Help for the Caring

Help for the Caring

◆

a Bibliography and Filmography for Family Caregivers of Alzheimer's Patients

Brenda Parris Sibley

Writers Club Press
New York   Lincoln   Shanghai

Help for the Caring
a Bibliography and Filmography for Family Caregivers of Alzheimer's Patients

Writers Club Press
an imprint of iUniverse, Inc.

For information address:
iUniverse
2021 Pine Lake Road, Suite 100
Lincoln, NE 68512
www.iuniverse.com

ISBN: 0-595-25356-3 (Pbk)
ISBN: 0-595-65119-4 (Cloth)

Printed in the United States of America

Always in memory of my mother, Jessie Lee Parris,
1916-1996, a victim of Alzheimer's Disease

and in honor of my sister and brother-in-law,
Myrtle and Simeon Allen,
my partners in caring for my mother

Contents

Preface

My idea for this book began with my Web site, *A Year to Remember...with My Mother and Alzheimer's Disease* (URL: *http://www.zarcrom.com/users/yeartorem/*) as I added a brief bibliography and filmography along with my journal, poems, photos of my mother, and links to Alzheimer's resources on the Internet. Just as the site grew from a handful of pages to over 400, so the bibliography and filmography grew gradually, bit by bit.

In searching the literature, I have not found a bibliography of Alzheimer's that has been published since the 1980s. I have not found bibliographies in publication that have been complied just for the family caregiver. Neither have I found a bibliography that covered Alzheimer's in fiction, poetry, or children's books. The addition of a filmography, appendixes covering Web resources, and Alzheimer's Association chapters, I believe will make this a valuable book for family caregivers and support groups.

I began the bibliography in 1996 with the books I had read while I was my mother's caregiver. Soon my career as a librarian influenced my seeking out more additions to the bibliography and filmography through my own network's catalog (Library Management Network, Decatur, AL), through other library catalogs that began to appear on the Web, including those of the Library of Congress and OCLC (Online Computer Library Center).

In the past year, every time I have thought the bibliography/filmography was complete and ready to publish, I would discover more books and videos. With the help of new technologies and print-on-demand publishers like iUniverse, publishing is booming, and authors have greater opportunities than ever before. Thus, this book will no doubt be slightly out of date as soon as it is published.

Keeping it up to date can be an ongoing project, and I can foresee the possibility of many future editions.

When available, ISBNs have been added in order to aid in locating and purchasing books. Also, when available, authors' Web site URLs (Uniform Resource Locators) have been included. Note that URLs may change at any time, and some may not be valid even by the time this book is published. If a URL does not work, it may help, beginning at the right, to back off the address to the preceding slash (/), successively, in an attempt to discover the valid URL. Please note that not all URLs have "www" as a part of the address.

Any omitted or additional publications or productions may be e-mailed to me at *bpsibley@mindspring.com* for inclusion in the next edition.

Acknowledgements

I would like to thank Dorothy Womack who got me going on this book on which I had been procrastinating. Dorothy and I are publishing with iUniverse at the same time and helping one another along. I would like to thank Kathleen Newton, my former Managing Editor at Suite 101, for helping me to believe I can write about this disease more widely than just about my own personal experience with caregiving. Thanks also to so many others I have met on the Internet who have believed in me and my ability to share what I have learned about Alzheimer's. Thanks to my siblings for being there with me through my caregiving experience, for being partners with me in caring. And thanks to my agent, editor, accountant husband, Richard, for proofreading, making corrections and suggestions, for attending to my bookkeeping, and for telling me back in 1996, just after my mother's death, that I needed to write about it to get my emotions onto paper and into a computer and to share it with others so that I myself could begin to heal.

Introduction

This bibliography and filmography covers mainly books written or films produced for caregivers and other family members of Alzheimer's patients. Books written for medical professionals have been omitted, although there may be some overlap, including some books that may have originally been intended for geriatric nurses or social workers. Books of research have been omitted other than a few popular titles. Theses and dissertations have been omitted. Although some might be of interest to general caregivers, they are not normally available to them except at university research libraries.

The chapters on poetry, fiction, children's books, and film attempt to compile everything written or produced which has an Alzheimer's victim as a character. These have not all been read or reviewed, thus the content or view taken is not necessarily that of the author. The chapter on film mixes both fiction and nonfiction, as does the chapter of children's literature, making no attempt to separate popular movies from educational films.

No attempt has been made to determine if books included are still in print. Even if they are not in print, they have value in a bibliography as they may be available in libraries as well as from out-of-print dealers. The final appendix lists book sources, including out-of-print dealers, and library catalogs on the Web, including the catalog of the Benjamin B. Green-Field Library at The Alzheimer's Association.

It is my hope that this bibliography and filmography will be the first of many editions that will be useful to family caregivers, early onset Alzheimer's patients, support group leaders, librarians, authors, and geriatric nurses and social workers.

1

Books about Alzheimer's and Caregiving

Abrignani, Catherine A. *Alzheimer's Disease: Activities That Work.* Bossier City, LA: Professional Printing & Publishing, 1991. ISBN: 1877735345

Activity Programming for Persons with Dementia: a Sourcebook. Chicago: Alzheimer's Association, 1995.

Adams, Martha O. *Alzheimer's Disease: a Call to Courage for Caregivers.* St. Meinard, IN: Abbey Press, 1986. ISBN: 0870292021

Aisen, Paul S. *Alzheimer's Disease: Questions and Answers.* Basingstoke, Hampshire, England; Coral Springs, FL: Merit Publishing International, 1997. ISBN: 187341336X

Alterra, Aaron. *The Caregiver: a Life with Alzheimer's.* South Royalton, VT: Steerforth Press, 1999. ISBN: 1883642620

Alzheimer Disease: a Handbook for Care. Toronto: Alzheimer Society of Canada, 1991. ISBN: 0969530102.

Alzheimer Journey: the Road Ahead. Modules 1 and 2. Toronto: Alzheimer Society of Canada, 1998.

Alzheimer's Disease: a Guide for Families and Other Caregivers, edited by Lenora S. Powell. 3rd ed. Cambridge, MA: Perseus Pub., 2002. ISBN: 0738205982

Alzheimer's Disease: a Handbook for Caregivers. St. Louis: Mosby, 1998. ISBN: 0815126069

Antonangeli, Judith M. *Of Two Minds: a Guide to the Care of People with the Dual Diagnosis of Alzheimer's Disease and Mental Retardation.* Malden, MA: Cooperative for Human Services, 1995.

Aronson, Miriam K. *Understanding Alzheimer's Disease: What it Does, How to Cope with it, Future Directions.* New York: Charles Scribner, 1988. ISBN: 0684184753

At Home with Alzheimer's Disease: Useful Adaptations to the Home Environment. Rev. ed. Ottawa: Canada Mortgage and Housing Corporation, 1990. ISBN: 0662579879

Bair, Frank E. *Alzheimer's, Strokes, and 29 Other Neurological Disorders Sourcebook: Basic Information for the Layperson.* Detroit, MI: Omnigraphics, 1993. ISBN: 1558887482

Bastedo, Deborah A. *Make a Difference...a Practical Approach to Dementia Care.* Bloomington, IN: 1stBooks Library, 2002. ISBN: 0759683174

Batiuk, Tom and Chuck Ayers. *Safe Return Home: an Inspirational Book for Caregivers of Alzheimer's.* Kansas City, MO: Andrews McMeel Pub., 1998. ISBN: 0836269136

Beasley, Edward D. *Alzheimer's Disease "Fighting For Financial Survival": a Financial and Legal Guide to Economic Survival for Alzheimer's Patients and Their Families.* Hearth Publishers, 2000. ISBN: 1889902152

Beerman, Susan. *Eldercare 911: The Caregiver's Complete Handbook for Making Decisions.* Amherst, NY: Prometheus Books, 2002. ISBN: 159102014X

Bell, Virginia. *The Best Friend's Approach to Alzheimer's Care*. Baltimore, MD: Health Professions Press, 1996. ISBN: 1878812351

Blessed Are the Caregivers: Practical Advice and Encouragement for Those Providing Care to Others, edited by Bob Russell, Danny Cain, Barrett Shaw. Prospect, KY: NB Publishing & Marketing, 1995. ISBN: 0964663007

Bornstein, Robert F. *When Someone You Love Needs Nursing Home, Assisted Living, or In-Home Care: the Complete Guide*. New York: Newmarket Press, 2002. ISBN: 1557045348

Bowlby, Carol. *Therapeutic Activities with Persons Disabled by Alzheimer's Disease and Related Disorders*. Gaithersburg, MD: Aspen, 1993.

Brackey, Jolene. *Creating Moments of Joy for the Person with Alzheimer's or Dementia: a Journal for Caregivers*. West Lafayette, IN: Purdue University Press, 2000. ISBN: 1557532125

Brawley, Elizabeth C. *Designing for Alzheimer's Disease: Strategies for Creating Better Care Environments*. New York: John Wiley, 1997. ISBN: 0471139203

Bridges, Barbara J. *Therapeutic Caregiving: a Practical Guide for Caregivers of Persons with Alzheimer's and Other Dementia Causing Diseases*. Mill Creek, WA: BJB Pub., 1996. ISBN: 0964517809 URL: *http://pages.prodigy.net/bjbservices/* (See Chapter 10, Reviews of Selected Books.)

Calkins, Margaret P. *Design for Dementia: Planning Environments for the Elderly and the Confused*. Owings Mill, MD: National Health Pub., 1988.

Calkins, Margaret P. *Key Elements of Dementia Care: Alzheimer's / Dementia Care Focus*. Chicago: Alzheimer's Association, 1997.

A Caregiver's Guide to Nutrition and Feeding. New York: The Western New York Chapter of the Alzheimer's Association.

Caring for Alzheimer's Patients: a Guide for Family and Healthcare Providers, edited by Gary D. Miner. New York: Plenum Press, 1989. ISBN: 0306431998

Caring for an Alzheimer's Patient across the Miles. Rockville, MD: American Health Assistance Foundation, 1987.

Caring for the Caregiver: a Guide to Living with Alzheimer's Disease. Morris Plains, NJ: Parke-Davis, 1994.

Caron, Wayne A. *Alzheimer's Disease: the Family Journey*. Plymouth, MN: North Ridge Press, 2001. ISBN: 0962961426

Carroll, David L. *When Your Loved One Has Alzheimer's*. New York: Harper & Row, 1990. ISBN: 0060916672

Cassistre, Debra. *Activity Ideas for the Budget Minded*. Forest Knolls, CA: Elder Books, 1994. ISBN: 0943873053

Castleman, Michael. *There's Still a Person in There: the Complete Guide to Treating and Coping With Alzheimer's*. New York: Perigee, 2000. ISBN: 0399526358.

Cayton, Harry. *Alzheimer's At Your Fingertips: the Comprehensive Dementia Reference Book for the Year 2000*. London: Class Publishing, 1997. ISBN: 1872362710

Charker, Jan. *Forget-Me-Not: Caring for an Alzheimer Patient*. Rozelle, NSW: Milner, Sally Publishing, 1994. ISBN: 1863511253

Check, William A. *Alzheimer's Disease*. New York: Chelsea House, 1989. (Encyclopedia of Health.) ISBN: 0791000567

Clayton, Shirley Anne. *Through My Eyes: a One on One Guide for Those Who Care for Loved Ones with Alzheimer's Disease*. Cottonwood, CA: Summerbreeze Publishers, 1997. ISBN: 0963224727

Cohen, Donna. *The Loss of Self: a Family Resource for the Care of Alzheimer's Disease and Related Disorders.* Revised and updated ed. New York: Norton, 2001. ISBN: 0393050165

Cohen, Elwood. *Alzheimer's Disease: Prevention, Intervention, and Treatment.* Los Angeles: NTC Contemporary, 1999. ISBN: 0879839643

Cohen, Uriel. *Holding on to Home: Designing Environments for People with Dementia.* Baltimore, MD: Johns Hopkins University Press, 1991.

Cordry, Cindy. *Hidden Treasures: Music & Memory Activities for People with Alzheimer's.* Eldersong Publication, 1994. ISBN: 1879633183

Coughlan, Patricia Brown. *Facing Alzheimer's: Family Caregivers Speak.* Lincoln, NE: Author's Guild/iUniverse, 2000. ISBN: 0595008038

Cutler, Neal R. *Understanding Alzheimer's Disease.* Jackson: University Press of Mississippi, 1996. ISBN: 0878059105; 0878059113

Davidson, Frena Gray. *Alzheimer's Frequently Asked Questions, Making Sense of the Journey.* Los Angeles: Lowell House, 1998. ISBN: 1565657888

Davidson, Frena Gray. *The Alzheimer's Sourcebook for Caregivers.* 3rd ed. Los Angeles: Lowell House, 1999. ISBN: 0737301317

Davidson, Frena Gray. *The Caregiver's Sourcebook.* Chicago: McGraw-Hill Professional, 2002. ISBN: 0737301368

Davidson, Frena Gray. *When Your Parent Has Alzheimer's.* Philadelphia: Xlibris, 2000. ISBN: 0738853216

Davies, Helen P. *Alzheimer's: the Answers You Need.* Forest Knolls, CA: Elder Books, 1998. ISBN: 0943873460

Delson, Sandra. *What to Do When Your Loved One Has Alzheimer's: a Guide for You.* Bayside, NY: Queensboro Community College, 1987.

Dippel, Raye Lynne. *Caring for the Alzheimer Patient: a Practical Guide*. 3rd ed. Buffalo, NY: Prometheus Books, 1996. ISBN: 1573921084

Dodds, Monica. *Caring for Your Aging Parent: a Guide for Catholic Families*. Huntington, IN: Our Sunday Visitor, 1997. ISBN: 087973731X

Dowling, James R. *Keeping Busy: a Handbook of Activities for Persons with Dementia*. Baltimore: Johns Hopkins University Press, 1995. ISBN: 0801850592 (paperback); 0801850584 (hardback)

Driscoll, Eileen Higgins. *Alzheimer's: a Handbook for the Caretaker*. Boston: Branden Books, 1994. ISBN: 0828319626

Dudding, Shirlee D. *Beyond the Wrinkles: Inspiration from a Nursing Home*. San Jose: Writer's Club Press / iUniverse, 2000.

Dunn, Hank. *Hard Choices for Loving People: CPR, Artificial Feeding, Comfort Care, and the Patient with a Life-threatening Illness*. 4th ed. Herndon, VA: A & A Publishers, 2001. ISBN: 1928560032

Eaker, Lorena Shell. *One Step at a Time: a Definitive Study of Alzheimer's Disease and a Practical Guide for Caregivers*. Church Hill, TN: SCK Publications, 1996. ISBN: 0965300005

Edwards, Allen Jack. *When Memory Fails: Helping the Alzheimer's and Dementia Patient*. New York: Perseus Publishing, 1994. ISBN: 0306446480

Entwistle, Charles C. *"I'm Just Not Myself Anymore": a Family Guide to Alzheimer's Disease*. Salt Lake City, UT: Northwest Publishing, 1994. ISBN: 1880416727

Everett, Deborah. *Forget Me Not: the Spiritual Care of People with Alzheimer's*. Edmonton, Alberta: Inkwell Press, 1996. ISBN: 0968046606.

Ewing, Wayne. *Tears in God's Bottle: Reflections on Alzheimer's Caregiving*. Tucson, AZ: Whitestone Circle Press, 1999. ISBN: 0966754700

Fabiano, Len. *Preventing Alzheimer Aggression: Supportive Therapy in Action, Book Two.* Seagrave, ON: Fabiano Consulting Services. ISBN 096955849X.

Family Care Guide. MA: The Alzheimer's Association of Eastern Massachusetts, 1988.

Feil, Naomi. *The Validation Breakthrough: Simple Techniques for Communicating with People with "Alzheimer's-type Dementia".* 2nd ed. Baltimore: Health Professions Press, 2002. ISBN: 1878812815

Fish, Sharon. *Alzheimer's: Caring for Your Loved Ones, Caring for Yourself.* Wheaton, IL: Harold Shaw Publishers, 1996. ISBN: 087788014X

Fitzray, B. J. *Alzheimer's Activities: Hundreds of Activities for Men and Women With Alzheimer's Disease and Related Disorders.* Windsor, CA: Rayve Productions. ISBN: 1877810800

Forrest, Deborah A. *Symphony of Spirits: Encounters with the Spiritual Dimensions of Alzheimer's.* New York: St. Martin's Press, 2000. ISBN: 0312241011

Forsythe, Elizabeth. *The Mystery of Alzheimer's: a Guide for Carers.* London: Kyle Cathie, 1996. ISBN: 1856262200

Free, Betty. *Quiet Moments for Caregivers and Their Families.* Wheaton, IL: Tyndale House Pub, 2002. ISBN: 0842353771

Friedman, Miles. *Your Father Has Alzheimer's.* Baltimore: PublishAmerica, 2002. ISBN: 1591293103

Garratt, Sally. *Rethinking Dementia: an Australian Approach.* Melbourne: Ausmed Publications, 1995. ISBN: 0646238256

Gfeller, Kate. *Music Therapy Programming for Individuals with Alzheimer's Disease and Related Disorders.* Iowa City, IA: School of Music, The University of Iowa, 1995.

Gillick, Muriel R. *Tangled Minds: Understanding Alzheimer's Disease and Other Dementias.* New York: Dutton, 1998. ISBN: 0525941452 (hardback); 0452941452 (paperback)

Granet, Roger. *Is It Alzheimer's?: What To Do When Loved Ones Can't Remember What They Should.* New York: Avon, 1998. ISBN: 0380786362.

Grollman, Earl A. *When Someone You Love Has Alzheimer's: the Caregiver's Journey.* Boston: Beacon Press, 1996. ISBN: 0807027200 (cloth); 0807027219 (paperback)

Grubbs, William M. *In Sickness & in Health: Caring for a Loved One with Alzheimer's.* Forest Knolls, CA: Elder Books, 1997. ISBN: 0943873126

Gruetzner, Howard. *Alzheimer's: the Complete Guide for Families and Loved Ones.* 3rd ed. New York: Wiley, 2001. ISBN: 0471379670

Guidelines for Care. Toronto: Alzheimer Society of Canada, 1992. ISBN: 0969530129.

Guidelines for Dignity: Goals of Specialized Alzheimer's / Dementia Care in Residential Settings. Chicago: Alzheimer's Association, 1992.

Gwyther, Lisa P. *Steps to Success: Decisions about Help at Home for Alzheimer's Caregivers.* Washington, DC: AARP Andrus Foundation, 2002.

Haisman, Pam. *Alzheimer's Disease: Caregivers Speak Out: a Guide to Understanding, Caring, and Coping.* Fort Myers, FL: Chippendale House Publishers, 1998. ISBN: 0966227204. (See Chapter 10, Reviews of Selected Books.)

Hall, Elizabeth T. *Caring for a Loved One with Alzheimer's Disease: a Christian Perspective.* New York: Haworth Pastoral Press, 2000. ISBN: 0789008726

Hall, Geri. *As Memory Fades - The Caregivers Challenge Begins: Understanding and Coping with Problem Behaviors Related to Memory Loss: a Learning Guide.*

Scottsdale, AZ (13400 E. Shea Boulevard, Scottsdale, AZ 85259): Mayo Clinic, 1999.

Hammond, William G. *The Alzheimer's Legal Survival Guide*. Overland Park, KS: The Elder & Disability Law Firm, P.A., 2000. ISBN: 1889902144

Harris, Phyllis Braudy. *Men Giving Care: Reflections of Husbands and Sons*. New York: Garland Pub., 1997. ISBN: 0815317921

Haugk, Kenneth C. *Christian Caregiving: a Way of Life*. Minneapolis: Augsburg Press, 1984. ISBN: 0806621230

Hawksford, Diane A. *Alzheimer's Disease: the Face of Alzheimer's*. Minnetonka, MN: The Diagnostic Center of Learning Patterns, 2000. ISBN: 1891421069

Hay, Jennifer. *Alzheimer's & Dementia: Questions You Have - Answers You Need*. Allentown, PA: People's Medical Society, 1996. ISBN: 1882606574

Haymon, Sandra W. *My Turn: Caring for Aging Parents & Other Elderly Loved Ones: a Daughters Perspective*. Tallahassee, FL: Magnolia Productions, 2001. ISBN: 0965296504

Hellen, Carly R. *Alzheimer's Disease: Activity Focused Care*. 2nd ed. Boston: Butterworth-Heinemann, 1998. ISBN: 0750699086

Hendershott, Anne. *The Reluctant Caregivers: Learning to Care for a Loved One with Alzheimer's Disease*. Westport, CT: Bergin & Garvey, 2000. ISBN: 0897897110

Heston, Leonard. *The Vanishing Mind: a Practical Guide to Alzheimer's Disease and Other Dementias*. New York: W.H. Freeman, 1991. ISBN: 0716721317 (hardback) 0716721929 (paperback)

Hidden Treasures: Music & Memory Activities for People with Alzheimer's. Mt. Airy, MD: Eldersong Publication, 1994. ISBN: 1879633183

Hodgkinson, Liz. *Alzheimer's Disease: Your Questions Answered.* London: Ward Lock, 1995. ISBN: 0706374010

Hodgson, Harriet W. *The Alzheimer's Caregiver: Dealing with the Realities of Dementia.* Minneapolis, MN: Chronimed, 1998. ISBN: 156561125X

Hodgson, Harriet W. *Alzheimer's: Finding the Words.* Minneapolis, MN: Chronimed, 1995. ISBN: 1565610717 (See Chapter 10, Reviews of Selected Books).

Hoffman, Stephanie. *Comforting the Confused: Strategies for Managing Dementia.* 2nd ed. New York: Springer Pub. Co., 2000. ISBN: 0826112617

Hoffman, Stephanie. *Special Care Programs for People with Dementia.* Baltimore: Health Professions Press, 1996. ISBN: 1878812335

Home Safety for the Alzheimer's Patient. San Diego: University of California, 1989.

Horowitz, David A. *Memory Loss and Dementia.* New York: DK Publishing, 2000. ISBN: 0789452014

Horticultural Therapy and the Older Adult Population, edited by Suzanne E. Wells. New York: Haworth Press, 1997. ISBN: 0789000458

Irigoyen, Fructuoso. *Alzheimer's Disease: a Primer for Caregivers.* McAllen, TX: Don Quixote Editions, 2001. ISBN: 0970955804

Jenny, Selly. *Memories in the Making, A Program of Creative Art Expression for Alzheimer Patients.* Orange, CA: Alzheimer's Association of Orange County. (2540 N. Santiago Blvd. Orange, CA 92867).

Johnson, Veronica. *At the Crossroads.* Veronica Birdsong, 2000. ISBN: 0970023707

Jones, Moyra. *Gentlecare: Changing the Experience of Alzheimer's Disease in a Positive Way*. Point Roberts, WA: Hartley & Marks, 1999. ISBN: 0881791717

Jorm, A.F. *A Guide to the Understanding of Alzheimer's Disease and Related Disorders*. Washington Square, NY: New York University Press, 1987. ISBN: 0814741703

Just for You: For People Diagnosed with Alzheimer Disease. Toronto: Alzheimer Society of Canada.

Just the Facts and More. Chicago: Alzheimer's Association, 1992.

Kakugawa, Frances K. *Mosaic Moon: Caregiving through Poetry*. Watermark Publishing, 2002. ISBN: 0972093206

Karpinski, Marion. *Quick Tips for Caregivers*. Medford, OR: Healing Arts Communications, 2000. ISBN: 0965387399

Keck, David. *Forgetting Whose We Are: Alzheimer's Disease and the Love of God*. Nashville: Abingdon Press, 1996. ISBN: 0687020883

Kelly, Cornelius. *Alzheimer's Disease Handbook*. Basingstoke, Hampshire, England: Merit Publishing International, 2000. ISBN: 1873413378

Kindig, Mary Norton. *Coping with Alzheimer's Disease and Other Dementias*. San Diego, CA: Singular Pub.Group, 1993. (Coping With Aging Series.) ISBN: 1565930975

Kitwood, Tom. *Person to Person: a Guide to the Care of Those with Failing Mental Powers*. Whatakers Way, Loughton Essex, UK: Gale Centre Publications, 1992.

Knittweis, Jim. *Alzheimer Solutions: a Personal Guide for Caregivers*. Sausalito, CA: Lucid Press, 2002. ISBN: 0964618451

Kociol, Lori. *Alzheimer: a Canadian Family Resource Guide.* Toronto: McGraw-Hill Ryerson, 1989. ISBN: 0075497743.

Koester, Robert J. *The Lost Wanderer: a Guide to Finding the Wandering Alzheimer's Disease Subject.* DBS Productions, 1999. ISBN: 1879471167

Kuhn, Daniel. *Alzheimer's Early Stages: First Steps in Caring and Treatment.* Alameda, CA: Hunter House, 1999. ISBN: 0897932633 (hardback); 0897932625 (paperback)

Lebow, Grace. *Coping with Your Difficult Older Parent: a Guide for Stressed-Out Children.* New York: Avon Books, 1999. ISBN: 038079750X

Le Navenec, Carole-Lynne. *One Day at a Time: How Families Manage the Experience of Dementia.* Westport, CT: Auburn House / Greenwood Press, 1996. ISBN: 0865692572

Lokvig, Jytte. *Alzheimer's A to Z: Secrets to Successful Caregiving.* Santa Fe, NM: Endless Circle Press; 2002. ISBN: 0971039003

Lovelace, Ruth A. *It's Not My Fault: a Sensitive, Realistic & Candid Journey into Alzheimer's Disease. 1999.* ISBN: 096791910X

Loverde, Joy. *The Complete Eldercare Planner: Where to Start, Which Questions to Ask, and How to Find Help.* 2nd ed. New York: Times Books, 2000. ISBN: 0812932781

Lovette, Katie. *Caring for an Alzheimer's Patient at Home.* Los Angeles, CA: Health Information Press, 1999. ISBN: 1885987161

Lowe, Paula C. *Care Pooling: How to Get the Help You Need to Care for the Ones You Love.* San Francisco: Berrett Koehler, 1993. ISBN: 1881052168.

Lyman, Karen A. *Day In, Day Out with Alzheimer's: Stress in Caregiving Relationships.* Philadelphia: Temple University Press, 1993. ISBN: 1566390974 (hardback) 1566390982 (paperback)

McCann-Beranger, Judy. *A Caregiver's Guide for Alzheimer Disease and Other Dementias.* Charlottetown, PEI: Alzheimer Society of PEI. ISBN 0968749607

McCrea, James M. *Talking to Children and Teens about Alzheimer's Disease: a Question and Answer Guidebook for Parents, Teachers, and Caregivers.* Pittsburgh, PA: Generations Together, University of Pittsburgh, Center for Social and Urban Research, 1992.

McKim, Donald K. *God Never Forgets: Faith, Hope, and Alzheimer's Disease.* Louisville, KY: Westminister / John Knox, 1997. ISBN: 0664257046

McLeod, Beth Witrogen. *And Thou Shalt Honor: the Caregiver's Companion.* Emmaus, PA: Rodale, 2002. ISBN: 1579545580

McLeod, Beth Witrogen. *Caregiving: the Spiritual Journey of Love, Loss, and Renewal.* New York: John Wiley, 1999. ISBN 0471254088

Mace, Nancy L. *The 36-Hour Day.* 3rd ed. Baltimore: Johns Hopkins Univ., 1999. ISBN 0801861489 (hardback); 0801861497 (paperback) (See Chapter 10, Reviews of Selected Books.)

Mace, Nancy L. *Dementia Care: Patient, Family and Community.* Baltimore, MD: Johns Hopkins University Press, 1990. ISBN 0801838592

Markin, R. F. *Coping with Alzheimer's: The Complete Care Manual for Patients and Their Families.* Rev. and updated ed. Secaucus, NJ: Carol Pub. Group, 1998. ISBN 0806519622

Mayo Clinic on Alzheimer's Disease, edited by Ronald D. Petersen. Rochester, MN: Mayo Clinic, 2002. ISBN: 1893005224

Medina, John J. *What You Need to Know about Alzheimer's Disease.* New Harbinger Publishers, 1999. ISBN: 1572241276

Miller, Joan E. *Circle of Hope Resource Manual: a Guide for Congregations Assisting Dementia Families.* Charlotte, NC: Piedmont Chapter of the Alzheimer's Association, 1998.

Molloy, William. *Alzheimer's Disease.* Buffalo, NY: Firefly Books, 1998. ISBN: 1552092410

Molloy, William. *Caring for Your Parents in their Senior Years: a Guide for Grown-up Children.* Buffalo, NY: Firefly Books, 1998. ISBN: 1552092054

Moreno, H. J. *The A-Z of Alzheimer's Disease: a Caregiver's Guide & Planner.* Alzheimer's A to Z, 1995. ISBN: 0964496208

Morris, Virginia. *How to Care for Aging Parents.* New York: Workman, 1996. ISBN: 1563054353

My House is Not My Home: Practical Technology to Make the Home Safe and Manageable for Persons with Dementia. Toronto: Senior Care / Ontario Ministry of Community and Social Services, Program Technology Branch, 1990. ISBN: 0969502907

Naughtin, Gerry. *When I Grow Too Old to Dream: Coping with Alzheimer's Disease.* North Blackburn, Australia: Collins Dove, 1991. ISBN: 1863710752

Nekola, Pat. *An Alzheimer's Guide: Activities Issues for People Who Care.* Waukesha, WI: Applewood Ink, 2002. ISBN: 0966061098

Nelson, James Lindermann. *Alzheimers: Answers to Hard Questions for Families.* New York: Doubleday, 1996. ISBN: 0385485336

Nissenboim, Sylvia. *The Positive Interactions Program of Activities for People with Alzheimer's Disease.* Baltimore: Health Professions Press, 1998 ISBN: 1878812408

Oliver, Rose. *Coping with Alzheimer's: a Caregiver's Emotional Survival Guide.* New York: Dodd, Mead & Co., 1987. ISBN: 039608933X

Olsen, Richard. *Homes That Help: Advice from Caregivers for Creating a Supportive Home Environment.* Newark, NJ: New Jersey Institute of Technology Press, 1993.

Olshevski, Jodi L. *Stress Reduction for Caregivers*. Philadelphia, PA: Brunner / Mazel, 1999. ISBN: 0876309406

Ostuni, Elizabeth. *Getting Through: Communicating When Someone You Care For Has Alzheimer's Disease*. Vero Beach, FL: Speech Bin, 1991. ISBN: 0937857017

Panella, John. *Day Care Programs for Alzheimer's Disease and Related Disorders*. New York: Demos, 1987.

Parrent, Joanne. *Courage to Care: A Caregiver's Guide through Each Stage of Alzheimer's*. Indianapolis, IN: Alpha Books, 2001. ISBN: 0028642023

Perry, Angela. *The American Medical Association Guide to Home Caregiving*. New York: John Wiley, 2001. ISBN: 0471414093

The Person with Alzheimer's Disease: Pathways to Understanding the Experience, edited by Phyllis Braudy. Baltimore: Johns Hopkins Univ. Press, 2002. ISBN: 0801868777

Pollen, Daniel A. *Hannah's Heirs: the Quest for the Genetic Origins of Alzheimer's Disease*. Expanded ed. New York: Oxford Univ. Press, 1996. ISBN: 0195106520

Post, Stephen G. *The Moral Challenge of Alzheimer's Disease*. 2nd ed. Johns Hopkins University Press, 2000. ISBN: 0801864100

Rader, Joanne. *Individualized Dementia Care: Creative, Compassionate Approaches*. New York: Springer Pub. Co., 1995. ISBN: 0826187307

Rau, Marie T. *Coping with Communication Challenges in Alzheimer's Disease*. San Diego, CA: Singular Pub. Group, 1993. ISBN: 1879105764

Raymond, Florian. *Surviving Alzheimer's: a Guide for Families*. Forest Knolls, CA: Elder Books. ISBN: 0943873002

Reisberg, Barry. *A Guide to Alzheimer's Disease: for Families, Spouses, and Friends*. New York: Free Press, 1983. ISBN: 0029263700

Residential Care: a Guide for Choosing a New Home. Chicago: Alzheimer's Association, 1998.

Ripoch, Danielle. *Alzheimer Disease Communication Guide: the FOCUSED Program for Caregivers,* 1996.

Roberts, D. Jeanne. *Taking Care of Caregivers: for Families and Others Who Care for People with Alzheimer's Disease and Other Forms of Dementia*. Palo Alto, CA: Emeryville, CA: Bull Pub. Co.; Distributed in the U.S. by Publishers Group West, 1991. ISBN: 0923521097

Roberts, Joan D. *Caring for Those with Alzheimer's: a Pastoral Approach*. Staten Island, New York, NY: Alba House, 1991. ISBN: 081890593X

Robinson, Anne. *Understanding Difficult Behaviors: Some Practical Suggestions for Coping with Alzheimer's Disease and Related Illnesses*. Ypsilanti, MI: Geriatric Education Center of Michigan, 1992.

Roche, Lyn. *Coping with Caring: Daily Reflections for Alzheimer's Caregivers*. Forest Knolls, CA: Elder Books, 1996. ISBN: 0943873290

Rogers, Joseph. *Candle and Darkness: Current Research in Alzheimer's Disease*. Chicago, IL: Bonus Books, 1998. ISBN: 1566250951

Ronch, Judah L. *Alzheimer's Disease: a Practical Guide for Those Who Help Others*. New York: Continuum, 1989. ISBN: 0826405002

Rowe, Robert V. *Alzheimer's, Day Care, Nursing Homes and Medicaid*. Robert V. Rowe, 1999. ISBN: 0966984625

The Rush Manual for Caregivers, edited by Daniel Kuhn. 4th ed. Chicago: Rush Alzheimer's Disease Center, 1999.

Safford, Florence. *Caring for the Mentally Impaired Elderly: a Family Guide.* New York: Henry Holt, 1987. ISBN: 0805000801

San Pietro, Mary Jo. *Successful Communication with Alzheimer's Disease Patients.* 1997.

Schiff, Myra. *Alzheimer: a Canadian Family Resource Guide.* Toronto: McGraw-Hill Ryerson, 1989. ISBN: 0075497743

Selby, Lynne. *Flowers for Mother: an A-Z Guide for Caregivers Coping with Alzheimer's Disease.* Santa Barbara: Capra Press, 1991.

Shenk, David. *The Forgetting: Alzheimer's: Portrait of an Epidemic.* New York: Doubleday, 2001. ISBN: 0385498373

Sheridan, Carmel. *Failure-Free Activities for the Alzheimer's Patient: a Guide for Caregivers.* New York: Dell, 1995. ISBN: 0440506050 (See Chapter 10, Reviews of Selected Books.)

Sheridan, Carmel. *Reminiscence: Uncovering a Lifetime of Memories.* San Francisco: Elder Books, 1991. ISBN: 094387310X

Sherman, James R. *Coping with Caregiver Worries.* Golden Valley, MN: Pathway Books, 1998 (Caregiver Survival Series.) ISBN: 0935538208

Sherman, James R. *Creative Caregiving.* Golden Valley, MN: Pathway Books, 1994 (Caregiver Survival Series.) ISBN: 0935538178

Sherman, James R. *The Magic of Humor in Caregiving.* Golden Valley, MN: Pathway Books, 1995 (Caregiver Survival Series.) ISBN: 0935538194

Sherman, James R. *Positive Caregiver Attitudes.* Golden Valley, MN: Pathway Books, 1994 (Caregiver Survival Series.) ISBN: 0935538186

Sherman, James R. *Preventing Caregiver Burnout.* Golden Valley, MN: Pathway Books, 1994 (Caregiver Survival Series.) ISBN: 093553816X

Siciliano, Paula. *Caring for the Person with Alzheimer's or Other Dementias.* Rev. ed. Albuquerque, NM: Hartman Publishing, 1999. ISBN: 1888343346

Silverstein, Nina M. *Dementia and Wandering Behavior: Concern for the Lost Elder.* New York: Springer Publishing, 2002. ISBN: 0826142621

Smith, Fred. *Alzheimer's, Dementia & Memory Loss.* TOP, 2003. ISBN: 0970368453

Snowden, David. *Aging With Grace: What the Nun Study Teaches Us About Leading Longer, Healthier, and More Meaningful Lives.* New York: Bantam Doubleday Dell, 2002. ISBN: 0553380923

Souren, Liduïn. *Broken Connections: Part 1, Origin and Course, the World of the Patient: Alzheimer's Disease.* Lisse: Berwyn, PA: Swets & Zeitlinger Publishers, 1994. ISBN: 9026513348

Souren, Liduïn. *Broken Connections: Part 2, Practical Guidelines for Caring for the Alzheimer Patient.* Lisse: Berwyn, PA: Swets & Zeitlinger Publishers, 1994. ISBN: 9026513712

Steps for Caregivers: Caring for Persons with Alzheimer's Disease. Chicago: Alzheimer's Association, 1999.

Stokes, Graham. *Challenging Behaviour in Dementia: a Person-Centred Approach.* Bicester: Speechmark Publishing Ltd., 2000. ISBN: 0863882501

Stoller, Shirley. *Hug and Hold Hands: Handbook of Wit and Wisdom for Caregivers of Alzheimer's Disease.* 2nd ed. San Diego, CA: San Diego Writers' Monthly Press, 2000. ISBN: 188551607X

Strauss, Claudia J. *Talking to Alzheimer's: Simple Ways to Connect When You Visit with a Family Member or Friend.* Oakland, CA: New Harbinger, 2002. ISBN: 1572242701

Strecker, Teresa R. *Alzheimer's: Making Sense of Suffering.* Lafayette, LA: Vital Issues Press, 1997. ISBN: 1563841339

Stones, Michael. *Alzheimer's Disease and Aggression*. North York, ON: Captus Press, 1997. ISBN: 1896691358

Strom, Kay Marshall. *A Caregiver's Survival Guide: How to Stay Healthy When Your Loved One Is Sick*. Downers Grove, IL: InterVarsity Press, 2000. ISBN: 0830822305

Tame, Amiria Choukair. *Healing the Wounds of Alzheimer's Disease*. Findlay, OH: DocuMall, 1999. ISBN: 0967218500

Tanner, Fredricka. *Caring: a Family Guide to Managing the Alzheimer's Patient at Home*. New York: New York City Alzheimer's Resource Center, 1985.

Tanzi, Rudy. *Decoding Darkness: the Search for the Genetic Causes of Alzheimer's Disease*. Cambridge, MA: Perseus Publishing, 2000. ISBN: 0738205265

Tebb, Susan Steiger. *Coping Successfully: Cognitive Strategies for Older Caregivers*. New York: Garland, 1995. ISBN: 0815319983

Teitel, Rosette. *The Handholder's Handbook: a Guide to Caregivers of People with Alzheimer's or Other Dementias*. New Brunswick, NJ: Rutgers University Press, 2001. ISBN: 0813529395; 0813529409 (paperback)

Thorsheim, Howard I. *I Remember When: Activity Ideas to Help People Reminisce*. Forest Knolls, CA: Elder Books, 2000. ISBN: 0943873177

A Time to Share: Activities for an Individual with Alzheimer's Disease. Green Bay, WI: Northeastern Wisconsin Chapter, Alzheimer's Association, 1993.

Tough Issues: Ethical Guidelines. Toronto: Alzheimer Society of Canada, 1996.

Twitchell, Karen L. *A Caregiver's Journey: Finding Your Way*. San Jose: Writer's Club Press / iUniverse, 2001. ISBN: 0595168353

Walters, Ginny Gordon. *Well Aged: Dining with Dignity*. Mill Valley, CA: GWhizz Books, 2001. ISBN: 0971313903

Warner, Mark. *The Complete Guide to Alzheimer's-Proofing Your Home*. West Lafayette, IN: Purdue University Press, 1998. ISBN: 1557531277

Watson, Bridget. *Music, Movement, Mind & Body*. Forest Knolls, CA: Elder Books, 1995. ISBN: 0943873363

Wenrick, Neta. *So Much More Than a Sing-A-Long*. Forest Knolls, CA: Elder Books, 1996. ISBN: 094387338X

Wexler, Nancy. *Mama Can't Remember Anymore: Care Management of Aging Parents and Loved Ones*. Thousand Oaks, CA: Wein & Wein Publishers, 1996. ISBN: 0962935824

Where to Begin: Living with Alzheimer Disease. Toronto: Alzheimer Association of Ontario, 1990.

Wolf-Klein, Gisèle P. *Keys to Understanding Alzheimer's Disease*. Hauppauge, NY: Barron's Educational Series, 1991. ISBN: 0812047583

Worship Services for People with Alzheimer's Disease and Their Families: A Handbook. Troy, NY: Eddy Alzheimer's Services; Albany, NY: Northeastern New York Chapter of the Alzheimer's Association.

Yale, Robyn. *Developing Support Groups for Individuals with Early Stage Alzheimer's Disease*. Baltimore: Health Professions Press, 1995. ISBN: 1878812262

Yale, Robyn. *Early Stage Alzheimer's Patient Support Groups: Research, Practice and Training Materials*. San Francisco: Special Projects Press, 1994.

Yale, Robyn. *A Guide to Facilitating Support Groups for Newly Diagnosed Alzheimer Patients*. Palo Alto, CA: Alzheimer's Association, Greater San Francisco Bay Area Chapter, 1991.

Zarit, Steven H. *The Hidden Victims of Alzheimer's Disease: Families under Stress*. New York: New York University Press, 1985. ISBN: 0814796621 (hardback); 081479663X (paperback)

Zgola, Jitka M. *Care That Works: a Relationship Approach to Persons with Dementia*. Baltimore: Johns Hopkins University Press, 1999. ISBN: 0801860253 (hardback); 0801860261 (paperback)

Zgola, Jitka M. *Doing Things: a Guide to Programming Activities for Persons with Alzheimer's Disease and Related Disorders*. Baltimore: Johns Hopkins University Press, 1987. ISBN: 080183466X (hardback); 0801834678 (paperback)

2

Biographies and Personal Stories

Alterra, Aaron. *The Caregiver: a Life with Alzheimer's*. South Royalton, VT: Steerforth Press, 2000. ISBN: 1586420070

Anifantaskis, Harry. *The Diminished Mind: the Jean Tyler Story*. Blue Ridge Summit, PA: Tab Books, 1991. ISBN: 0830634657

Apperson, Bob. *My Mother's Keeper: a Middle-Aged Son's Experiences as Caregiver for His Alzheimer-Afflicted Mother*. Authority Press Inc., 2001. ISBN: 1929059108

Artley, Bob. *Ginny: a Love Remembered*. Ames, IA: Iowa State Univ. Press, 1993. ISBN: 0813821045

Atkins, Marguerite Henry. *Also My Journey: a Personal Story of Alzheimer's*. Wilton: Morehouse-Barlow, 1985. ISBN: 0819213624

Avadian, Brenda. *Finding the Joy in Alzheimer's: Caregivers Share the Joyful Times*. Lancaster, CA: North Star Books, 2001. ISBN: 0963275224

Avadian, Brenda. *"Where's My Shoes?": My Father's Walk through Alzheimer's*. Lancaster, CA: North Star Books, 1999. ISBN: 0963275216

Barkman, Lorlie. *Remember, Dad? A Journey into Memory Loss*. Manitoba: Kindred Productions, 1999. ISBN: 0921788614

Baurys, Florence. *A Time for Alzheimer's: a True Story*. Houston, TX: Emerald Ink Pub., 1998. ISBN: 1885373139

Bayley, John. *Elegy for Iris*. New York: St. Martin's Press, 1999. ISBN: 0312198647

Bayley, John. *Iris and Her Friends: a Memoir of Memory and Desire*. New York: W.W. Norton, 2000. ISBN: 039304856X

Bell, Sherry M. *Visiting Mom: an Unexpected Gift*. Sedonia, AZ: Elder Press, 2000. ISBN: 0967708109

Blank, Louis. *Alzheimer's Challenged & Conquered?* London: Foulsham, 1995. ISBN: 0572021968

Boden, Christine. *Who Will I Be When I Die?* North Blackburn, Victoria, Australia: HarperCollins Religious, 1998. ISBN: 1863717331

Boggs, J. Robert. *I'll Move Over: Spouse and Family Stress in Dealing with Alzheimer's*. 3rd ed. Winona Lake, IN: Boggs' Books, 1994. ISBN: 0964888017

Bristow, Lois. *Will I Be Next? the Terror of Living with Familial Alzheimer's Disease: Bea Gorman's Life Story*. Acampo, CA: Hope Warrne Press, 1996. ISBN: 0964888505

Brown, Audrey. *A Matter of Timing: Alzheimer's, a Carer's Journey*. Lewes: Book Guild, 1998. ISBN: 1857763319

Brown, Dorothy S. *Handle with Care: a Question of Alzheimer's*. Buffalo, NY: Prometheus Books, 1984. ISBN: 0879752718 (hardback); 0932910475 (paperback)

Burchett, Harold Ewing. *Last Light: Staying True through the Darkness of Alzheimer's*. Colorado Springs: NavPress, 2002. ISBN: 1576832988

Caldwell, Marianne. *Gone without a Trace*. Forest Knolls, CA: Elder Books, 1995. (See Chapter 10, Reviews of Selected Books.)

Callahan, Sally. *My Mother's Voice*. Forest Knolls, CA: Elder Books, 1998. ISBN: 0943873495

Cassel, Franklin K. *Flowers for Peggy*. Lancaster, PA. (Brethren Village, P. O. Box 5093): F. Cassel, 1997.

Childress, Ellen. *Shattered Lives: Finding Hope in the Midst of Alzheimer's and Other Related Dementia*. Pittsburgh, PA: Dorrance Publishing, 2000. ISBN: 0805948120

Clarke, Eunice A. *When Mother Came to Live: Coping With Alzheimer's*. Bloomington, IN: 1stBooks Library, 2002. ISBN: 0759696837

Cloud, Marie. *Stolen Memories: One Family's Experience with Alzheimer's Disease*. San Jose: Writer's Club Press / iUniverse, 2001. ISBN: 0595158498

Combs, Linda. *A Long Goodbye*. Winston-Salem, NC: Combs Publishing, 1994.

Combs, Linda. *A Long Goodbye and Beyond: Coping with Alzheimer's*. Wilsonville, OR: Book Partners, 1998. ISBN: 1885221835

Confer, Grayce Bonham. *Alzheimer's: Another Opportunity to Love*. Kansas City, MO: Beacon Hill Press, 1992. ISBN: 0834114038

Cooney, Eleanor. *Death in Slow Motion: My Mother's Descent into Alzheimer's*. New York: HarperCollins. 2003. ISBN: 0066213967

Copeman-High, Barbara. *Elsie's Silent Cries*. Ontario: B. Copeman-High, 2000. ISBN: 0920439381

Curtman, Rose Marie. *My Renaissance: a Widow's Healing Pilgrimage to Tuscany*. Sterling, VA: Capital Books, 2002. ISBN: 1931868042

Danforth, Art. *Living with Alzheimer's: Ruth's Story: the Personal Story of Two Victims of Senile Dementia*. Falls Church, VA: Prestige Press, 1986.

Daniel, John. *Looking After: a Son's Memoir*. Washington, DC: Counterpoint Press, 1996. ISBN: 1887178597

Danna, Jo. *When Alzheimer's Hits Home*. Briarwood, NY: Palomino Press, 1995. ISBN: 0961003642

Darby, Jean. *I Still Love You: the Love Story of an Alzheimer's Caregiver*. Bloomington, IN: 1stBooks Library, 2001. ISBN: 0759620199

Darnell, Owen. *A Room Without Doors*. Ormond Beach, FL: Flagler Chapter Alzheimer's Association, 1995.

Davidson, Ann. *Alzheimer's, a Love Story: One Year in My Husband's Journey*. Secaucus, NJ: Carol Pub. Group, 1997. ISBN: 1559724188

Davis, Maggie Steincrohn. *Caring in Remembered Ways: the Fruit of Seeing Deeply*. Blue Hill, ME: Heartsong Books, 1999. ISBN: 0963881337

Davis, Patti. *Angels Don't Die: My Father's Gift of Faith*. New York: HarperCollins, 1995. ISBN: 0060173246

Davis, Patti. *A Long Goodbye*. New York: Alfred A. Knopf, 1997. ISBN: 0679450920

Davis, Robert. *My Journey into Alzheimer's Disease*. Wheaton, IL: Tyndale House, 1989. ISBN: 0875651534

Donahue, Sandie. *Fading Angel: a Chronicle of Love*. Banbury Publishing. ISBN: 0970600704

Dyer, Joyce. *In a Tangled Wood: an Alzheimer's Journey*. Dallas: Southern Methodist University Press, 1996. ISBN: 0870743961 (hardback); 087074397X (paperback)

Ellison, George Vernon. *She Never Said Goodbye: My Wife's Disappearance Down a Road of No Return - Alzheimer's*. Vista, CA: Aquarius House Press, 2000. ISBN: 1882888510 (hardback); 1882888529 (paperback)

Erb, Clinton A. *Losing Lou-Ann*. Brandon, VT: Holistic Education Press, 1996. ISBN: 0962723266

Ernaux, Annie. *I Remain in Darkness*. New York: Seven Stories Press, 2001. ISBN: 1583220143 (hardback); 1583220526 (paperback)

Forbis, Diane Dibb. *With Words That Once Were His: an Alzheimer's Experience*. Boise, ID: Legendary Publishing Co., 2000. ISBN: 1887747370

Forrest, Deborah A. *Symphony of Spirits: Encounters with the Spiritual Dimensions of Alzheimer's*. New York: St. Martin's Press, 2000. ISBN: 0312241011

Fournier, Christine. *On the Sunny Side of the Street: an Alzheimer's Journey*. Ednia, MN: Beaver's Pond Press, 2002. ISBN: 1931646163

Gamba, Louis F. *Natalina, Once So Bright*. Pittsburgh: CeShore Pub., 2000. ISBN: 1585010227

Gard, Robert Edward. *Beyond the Thin Line*. Madison, WI: Prairie Oak Press, 1992. ISBN: 1879483068

Goyder, Julie. *We'll Be Married in Fremantle: Alzheimer's Disease and the Everyday Act of Storying*. Fremantle, Western Australia: Fremantle Arts Center Press. 2001. ISBN: 1863683119

Granger, Persis R. *Shared Stories from Daughters of Alzheimer's: Writing a Path to Peace*. San Jose: Writer's Club Press / iUniverse, 2002. ISBN: 059522119X

Grant, Linda. *Remind Me Who I Am Again*. London: Granta Books, 1999. ISBN: 1862072442

Gray, David Dodson. *I Want to Remember: a Son's Reflection on His Mother's Alzheimer Journey*. Wellesley, MA: Roundtable Press, 1993. ISBN: 093451206X

Grubbs, William M. *In Sickness & in Health: Caring for a Loved one with Alzheimer's Disease*. Forest Knolls, CA: Elder Books, 1997. ISBN: 0943873126

Guerreno, Gene. *Love Meets Alzheimer's.* Rutledge Books, 2000. ISBN: 158244062X

Hamilton, Heidi. *Glimmers: a Journey into Alzheimer's Disease.* White Cloud Press, 2002. ISBN: 188399179X

Harrod, Lois Marie. *Spelling the World Backwards.* Aiken, SC: Palanquin Press, 2000. ISBN: 1891508059

Haugse, John E. *Heavy Snow: My Father's Disappearance into Alzheimer's.* Deerfield Beach, FL: Health Communications, 1999. ISBN: 1558746773

Heckman-Owen, Carol. *Life with Charlie: Coping with an Alzheimer Spouse or Other Dementia Patient and Keeping Your Sanity.* Ventura, CA: Pathfinder Pub., 1992. ISBN: 0934793417

Heinemann, Faith M. *A Different Reality: Alzheimer's Love Story.* CA: F. Heinemann, 2000. ISBN: 0966523431

Henderson, Cary Smith. *Partial View: an Alzheimer's Journal.* Dallas, TX: Southern Methodist University Press, 1998. ISBN: 0870744380

Heywood, Bernard. *Caring for Maria: an Experience of Successfully Coping with Alzheimer's Disease.* Rockport, MA: Element, 1994. ISBN: 1852305029

Hilden, Julie. *The Bad Daughter.* Chapel Hill, NC: Algonquin Books, 1998. ISBN: 1565121856

Holland, Gail Bernice. *For Sasha, with Love: an Alzheimer's Crusade: the Anne Bashkiroff Story.* New York: Dembner Books, 1985. ISBN: 0934878544

Honel, Rosalie Walsh. *Journey with Grandpa: Our Family's Struggle with Alzheimer's Disease.* Baltimore: Johns Hopkins University Press, 1988. ISBN: 0801837219

Jahraus, Cecil D. *Alice, Artas, and Alzheimer's.* Bismark, ND: C. Jahraus, 1995.

Jansen, Verna A. *Alzheimer's, the Good, the Sad & the Humorous: a Daughter's Story*. South Barre, MA: V. A. Jansen, 1999. ISBN: 0967256305

Kaylan, Amelia. *Don't Cry Alone*. Kingston, ON: A. E. Hogeboom, Brown & Martin, 1985. ISBN: 0969212607

Kidd-Madison, Nellie. *Living with John: Caring for a Loved One with Alzheimer's Disease*. Gretna, LA: Wellness Institute, 2000. ISBN: 1587410613

Knowles, Carrie. *The Last Childhood: a Family Story of Alzheimer's*. New York: Three Rivers Press, 2000. ISBN: 0609806483

Konek, Carol Wolfe. *Daddyboy: a Memoir*. St. Paul, MN: Graywolf Press, 1991. ISBN: 1555971539

Kraft, Frances A. *Fading: One Family's Journey with a Woman Silenced by Alzheimer's*. Detroit Lakes, MN: BL Publications, 2000. ISBN: 1890766143

Layton, Annamae Brinkman. *The Mind Inside Isn't Me: "Is It All For the Best?": Words Spoken from the Heart of Someone Who Had Alzheimer's*. Salem, OR: Annamae Layton, 1992.

Love is Ageless: Stories about Alzheimer's Disease, edited by Jessica Bryan. 2nd ed. Felton, CA: Lompico Creek Press, 2002. ISBN: 0961931116 URL: *http://www.loveisageless.com/*

McDonald, Diane. *To Pap with Love*. San Jose: Writer's Club Press / iUniverse, 2002. ISBN: 059522749X

McGowin, Diana Friel. *Living in the Labyrinth: a Personal Journey through the Maze of Alzheimer's*. New York: Delacorte Press, 1993. ISBN: 0786200669 (hardback); 0786200677 (paperback) (See Chapter 10, Reviews of Selected Books.)

McKiernan, Bernadette. *Talking to Myself: the Inspirational Journal of a Mad Caregiver*. B. McKiernan, 1998. ISBN: 0970982402

McQuilkin, J. Robertson. *A Promise Kept*. Wheaton, IL: Tyndale House, 1998. ISBN: 0842350993

Marcell, Jacqueline. *Elder Rage or, Take My Father... Please! How to Survive Caring for Aging Parents*. Impressive Press, 2001. ISBN: 0967970318 URL: *http://www.ElderRage.com* (See Chapter 10, Reviews of Selected Books.)

Markle, George V. *Donna's Story: the Tragedy of Alzheimer's*. NM: G. Markle.

Mathiasen, Patrick. *An Ocean of Time: Alzheimer's: Tales of Hope and Forgetting*. New York: Scribner, 1997. ISBN: 0684822520

Miller, Sue. *The Story of My Father: a Memoir*. New York: Alfred A. Knopf, 2003. ISBN: 0375414797

Mitchell, Marilyn. *Dancing on Quicksand: a Gift of Friendship in the Age of Alzheimer's*. Boulder: Johnson Books, 2002. ISBN: 1555663214

Moskowitz, Bette Ann. *Do I Know You?: Living through the End of a Parent's Life*. New York: Kodansha International, 1998. ISBN: 1568362102

Murphy, Beverly Bigtree. *He Used to Be Somebody: a Journey into Alzheimer's Disease through the Eyes of a Caregiver*. Boulder, CO: Gibbs Associates, 1995. ISBN: 0943909147 (See Chapter 10, Reviews of Selected Books.)

Murphy, Earline M. *Laughter Among the Tears: Living with Alzheimer's*. Shawnee, OK: Fly Away Press, 1998. ISBN: 0966546806

Peterson, Penny A. *Letters to My Aunt: an Alzheimer's Chronicle*. Sun Lakes, AZ: Desert State Publishing, 1997. ISBN: 0965596907

Pierce, Charles. *Hard To Forget: an Alzheimer's Story*. New York: Random House, 2000. ISBN: 0679452915

Rain, Mary Summer. *Love Never Sleeps: Living At Home with Alzheimer's*. Charlottesville, VA: Hampton Roads Publishing, 2002. ISBN: 1571743251

Rhodes, Cheryl. *Recipes My Mother Forgot: Family Style Cooking and a Caregiver's Guide to Alzheimer's Disease*. Surrey, BC: Mermaid-Rhodes Publishing, 2000. ISBN: 096864130X

Roach, Marion. *Another Name for Madness*. Boston: Houghton Mifflin, 1985. ISBN: 0395353734

Rose, Larry. *Show Me the Way to Go Home*. Forest Knolls, CA: Elder Books, 1996. ISBN: 0943873088 (See Chapter 10, Reviews of Selected Books.)

Roth, M. Joanne. *Thanks for the Memories: My Journey with Alzheimer's As a Caregiver to My Mother*. Pittsburgh: Dorrance Publishing Co., 2001. ISBN: 0805953213

Rowe, Robert V. *Alzheimer's (A Caregiver's Day-By-Day Account)*. Robert V. Rowe, Publisher, 1998. ISBN: 0966984609

Royer, Ruth S. *Sarah R. Royer: a Young Alzheimer's Patient: My Memory of Her*. New York: Vantage Press, 1991. ISBN: 053309187X

Rozelle, Ron. *Into that Good Night*. New York: Farrar, Straux and Giroux, 1998. ISBN: 0374177112

Schrantz, Joe. *Gladys: Love Conquers Alzheimer's*. Infinity Publishing, 2002. ISBN: 0741409682

Seegmiller, Judy. *Life with Big Al (Early Alzheimer's): a Caregivers Diary*. Provo, UT: Alexanders Publishing, 2000. ISBN: 157636108X

Seymour, Claire. *Precipice: Learning to Live with Alzheimer's Disease*. New York: Vantage Press, 1983. ISBN: 0533056195

Shanks, Lela Knox. *Your Name is Hughes Hannibal Shanks: a Caregiver's Guide to Alzheimer's*. Lincoln: University of Nebraska Press, 1996. ISBN: 080324245X

Sibley, Brenda Parris. *Waiting for the Morning: a Mother and Daughter's Journey through Alzheimer's Disease.* San Jose: Writer's Club Press / iUniverse.com, 2001. ISBN: 059518782X

Siegel, Frances. *Living with Alzheimer's Disease: One Couple's Journey.* Berkeley: Regent Press, 2000. ISBN: 1889059811

Simpson, Robert. *Through the Wilderness of Alzheimer's: a Guide in Two Voices.* Minneapolis, MN: Augsburg, 1999. ISBN: 0806638915

Smith, L. B. *Susie and Herman: a Story of Love and Caregiving.* Health Communications, 2002. ISBN: 1558749578

Smoller, Esther Strauss. *I Can't Remember: Family Stories of Alzheimer's Disease.* Philadelphia: Temple Univ. Press, 1997. ISBN: 1566395550 (hardback); 1566395569 (paperback)

Snyder, Lisa. *Speaking Our Minds: Personal Reflections from Individuals with Alzheimer's.* New York: W. H. Freeman, 1999. ISBN: 0716732246

Spohr, Betty Baker. *To Hold a Falling Star.* Seattle, WA: Storm Peak Press, 1995. ISBN: 096413571X (See Chapter 10, Reviews of Selected Books.)

Starkman, Elaine Marcus. *Learning to Sit in Silence.* Watsonville, CA: Papier-Mache Press, 1993. ISBN: 0918949432 (paperback); 0918949440 (hardback) (See Chapter 10, Reviews of Selected Books.)

Stone, Janet M. *My Parents and Alzheimer's: a Daughter's Story.* New York: Vantage Press, 2000. ISBN: 0533135516.

Turley, Jack. *Old Timers: a Son Witnesses His Mother's One-Way Journey into the Darkness of Alzheimer's Disease.* 1stBooks Library, 2002. ISBN: 0759674167

Twichell, Karen L. A *Caregiver's Journey: Finding Your Way.* San Jose: Writer's Club Press / iUniverse, 2001. ISBN: 0595168353

Upton, Rosemary Mason. *Glimpses of Grace: a Family Struggles with Alzheimer's*. Grand Rapids: Baker Book House, 1990. ISBN: 0801092094

Vogt, Kenneth. *Our Journey: Diary of a Caregiver*. Kansas City, MO: Beacon Hill Press, 1992. ISBN: 083411433X

Wall, Frank A. *Where Did Mary Go?: a Loving Husband's Struggle with Alzheimer's*. Amherst, NY: Prometheus Books, 1996. ISBN: 1573920703

Walsh, Mary B. *One Family's Journey through Alzheimer's*. Wheaton, IL: Tyndale House, 2000. ISBN 0842340956 (See Chapter 10, Reviews of Selected Books.)

Wheeler, Burton M. *Close to Me, But Far Away: Living with Alzheimer's*. Columbia, MO: University of Missouri Press, 2001. ISBN: 0826213804.

Wirsig, Woodrow. *I Love You, Too*. New York: M. Evans, 1990. ISBN: 0871316161.

Womack, Dorothy. *Passage into Paradise: the True Story of My Own Mother's Struggle with Alzheimer's Disease*. San Jose: Writer's Club Press / iUniverse, 2002. ISBN: 0595249264. (See Chapter 10, Reviews of Selected Books.)

Wright, Marian E. *With Love: a Caregiver's Journal*. San Jose: Writer's Club Press / iUniverse, 2000. ISBN: 0595091792

Young, Ellen P. *Between Two Worlds: Special Moments of Alzheimer's & Dementia*. Prometheus Books, 1999. ISBN: 1573926973

Zabbia, Kim Howes. *Painted Diaries: a Mother and Daughter's Experience through Alzheimer's*. Minneapolis: Fairview Press, 1996. ISBN: 157749007X (See Chapter 10, Reviews of Selected Books.)

Zeiger, Genie. *How I Find Her: a Mother's Dying and a Daughter's Life*. Santa Fe, NM: Sherman Asher Publishing, 2001. ISBN: 1890932167

3

Alzheimer's in Poetry

Abse, Dannie. "Alzheimer's." *Be Seated Thou: Poems*. Sheep Meadow Press, 2000, p. 86. ISBN: 187881883X

Bailey, Jan. "Alzheimer's." *Paper Clothes*. The Emrys Foundation, 1995, p. 12. ISBN: 0964577801

Block, Laurie. "Senile Dementia." *Prairie Fire*. v. 21, no. 1, Spring 2000, p. 156.

Booth, Phillip. "Fallback," *Literature & Aging: an Anthology*, edited by Martin Kohn, Carol Donley & Delese Wear. Kent, OH: Kent State University Press, 1992.

Bowers, Cathy Smith. "Alzheimer's." *Love That Ended Yesterday in Texas*. Texas Tech University Press, 1992. ISBN: 0896723011

Brown, Linda C. *Secret Waters*. Blue Begonia Press, 1997. (Women's Poetry Series.) ISBN: 0911287248

Calbert, Cathleen. "Listening to My Mother in the Alzheimer's Wing." *Poetry*. v. 178, no. 3, June 2001, p. 139.

Cherry, Kelly. "Alzheimer's." *Death and Transfiguration*. Louisiana State University Press, 1997.

Cirillo, Stacey, "As She Sits." *Alzheimer's Disease Caregivers Speak Out*, by Pam Haisman. Ft. Myers, FL: Chippendale House Publishers, 1998.

Clancy, Joseph P. *Ordinary Time*. Llandysul, Ceredigion, Wales: Gomer, 2000. ISBN: 1859027393

Davie, Donald. "Alzheimer's Disease for Kenneth Millar (Ross MacDonald)." *Collected Poems*. Chicago: University of Chicago Press, 1991. ISBN: 0226137619

Dyer, Paul B. *Please, Remember Me: Poems about Alzheimer's Disease*. Alzheimer's Association, 1995.

Eisenhart, Gail E. *Viola, Unstrung: an Alzheimer's Fugue*. Infinity Publishing, 2002. ISBN: 0741410362

Elkind, Sue Saniel. "Alzheimer's Patient." *San Fernando Poetry Journal*. v. 13, no. 4, 1990, p. 17.

Gay, Ross. "Alzheimer's." *The North American Review*. v. 286, no. 2, March-April 2001, p. 9.

Hacker, Mary. "Against Elegies." *Winter Numbers*. New York: Norton Press, 1995.

Ham, Jerry. *This Stranger in Our House*. Spokane, WA: The Inland Northwest Chapter of the Alzheimer's Association (720 W. Boone Ave., Suite 101, Spokane, WA 99201), 1999. (See Chapter 10, Reviews of Selected Books.)

Harrod, Lois Marie. *Spelling the World Backwards*. Palanquin Press, 2000. ISBN: 1891508059

Hart, Henry. "Alzheimer's." *The Rooster's Mask*. University of Illinois Press, 1998, p. 28. ISBN: 0252066928

Hicok, Bob. "Alzheimer's." *Southern Review*. v. 31, no. 2, Spring 1995, p. 41.

Kono, Juliet. "Elizabeth." *Tsunami Years*. Honolulu: Bamboo Ridge Press, 1995.

Larkin, Phillip. "The Old Fools." *Collected Poems*, edited by Anthony Thwaite. New York: Farrar, Straus & Giroux, 1989.

Louis, Adrian C. "Alzheimer's." *Ceremonies of the Damned*. University of Nevada Press, 1997, p. 37. ISBN 0874173027

MacDonald, Hugh. *Looking for Mother*. Windsor, ON: Black Moss Press, 1995. ISBN: 0887532594 (See Chapter 10, Reviews of Selected Books.)

Maylon, Carol. *Emma's Dead*. Toronto: Wolsak and Wynn, 1992. ISBN: 0919897312

Moreland, Margaret. "Alzheimer's Lesson." *Gift of Jade*. Forest Woods Media Productions, 1998. ISBN: 0938572210

Morgan, Betty. *Alzheimer's Alters Us All*. Lexington, VA: Betty Morgan, 1984.

O'Heir, Diane. "Shore." *Home Free*. New York: Atheneum, 1988.

Pepper, Leila. *In War with Time: Poems*. Windsor, ON: Black Moss Press, 1994.

Petrie, Paul. "Alzheimer's." *Kansas Quarterly*. v. 22, no.1-2, Winter-Spring 1990.

Rectenwald, Janet "Alzheimer's." *St. Anthony Messenger*. v. 108, no. 4, September 2000, p. 43.

Savard, Jeannine. "Alzheimer's." *The American Poetry Review*. v. 25, no. 2, March-April 1996, p. 42.

Schultz, Philip. "Alzheimer's." *Sixty Years of American Poetry*. New York: Henry N. Abrams, 1996.

Sierra, Sherry. "The Call." *The Writer*. v. 106, no. 3, March 1993, p. 23.

Silvermarie, Sue. *Tales from My Teachers on the Alzheimer's Unit*. Milwaukee, WI: Families International, 1996. ISBN: 087304293X

Smith Bower, Cathy. "Aphasia." *The Love That Ended Yesterday in Texas*. Lubbock, TX: Texas Tech University Press, 1993.

Sobsey, Cynthia. "Alzheimer." *Kalliope*. v. 16, no. 1, 1994, p. 22.

St. Andrews, B. A. (Bonnie) "Alzheimer's." *The Healing Muse*. Syracuse, NY: Silverman Reviews Press, 1999.

Wagoner, David. "Into the Nameless Places." *Broken Country: Poems*. Boston: Little, 1979.

Wallace, Ronald. "Alzheimer's." *The Uses of Adversity*. University of Pittsburgh Press, 1998.

Williams, William Kenneth. "Alzheimer's: the Husband." *Flesh and Blood*. Farrar Strauss Giroux, 1987. ISBN: 0374520909

Williams, William Kenneth. "Alzheimer's: the Wife." *Flesh and Blood*. Farrar Strauss Giroux, 1987. ISBN: 0374520909

Womack, Dorothy. *Alzheimer's Angels: a Compilation of Poetry Honoring Caregivers and Victims of Alzheimer's Disease*. San Jose: Writer's Club Press / iUniverse, 2002. ISBN: 0595245501

Young, Clemewell. "Alzheimer's." *Poets On*. v. 18, no. 2, Summer 1994, p. 37.

4

Alzheimer's in Fiction

Adderson, Caroline. *A History of Forgetting*. Toronto: Patrick Crean Editions, 1999. ISBN: 1894433017

Alba, Kathy A. *Concertos in D Major*. San Jose: Writer's Club Press / iUniverse, 2000 ISBN: 0595133339

Baer, Judy. *Libby's Story*. Wheaton, IL: Tyndale House Publishers, 2001. ISBN: 0842319239

Bernlef, J. *Out of Mind*. Translated by Adrienne Dixon. London: Faber, 1989.

Coyle, Beverly, J. *In Troubled Waters*. New York: Penguin, ISBN: 0140233016.

Delinsky, Barbara. *Shades of Grace*. New York: Harper & Collins, 1995. ISBN: 0060177810

Dorner, Marjorie. *Seasons of Sun and Rain*. Minneapolis: Milkweed Editions, 1999. ISBN: 1571310274

Drews, Bob. *Sandman*. San Jose, CA: Writers Club Press / iUniverse, 2001. ISBN: 0595206166

Dummer, Shirley. *Lost Love*. S. Dummer, 1994. ISBN: 0963347926

Fisher, Carrie. *Delusions of Grandmother*. New York: Simon & Schuster, 1994. ISBN: 0671882953

Frommer, Sara Hoskinson. *Witness in Bishop Hill: a Joan Spencer Mystery*. New York: St. Martin's Minotaur, 2002. ISBN: 0312302436

Goldman, Abe. *Holding on to Ettie*. Plantation, FL: Distinctive Pub. Corp., 1991. ISBN: 0942963105

Gordon, Mary. *The Rest of Life*. New York: Viking Press, 1993. ISBN: 0670838284

Haas, Cynthia. *Angel of Mercy: When a Loved One Has Alzheimer's*. AmErica House Book Publishers, 1999. ISBN: 1893162095

Hallinan, Timothy. *Incinerator*. New York: William Morrow & Co., 1992.

Harper, M.A. *The Worst Day of My Life, So Far: My Mother, Alzheimer's and Me*. Athens, GA: Hill Street Press, 2001. ISBN: 1892514974

Hegarty, Frances. *Let's Dance*. New York: Viking, 1995. ISBN: 0670866393

Ignatieff, Michael. *Scar Tissue*. New York: Farrar, Straus & Giroux, 1994. ISBN: 0374254281

Jennings, Kate. *Moral Hazard: a Novel*. New York: Fourth Estate, 2002. ISBN: 0007141084

Kingsolver, Barbara. *Animal Dreams*. New York: Scribner, 1991.

Lonergan, Kenneth. *The Waverly Gallery: A Play*. New York: Grove Press, 2000. ISBN: 0802137563

McBain, Ed. *Mischief: a Novel of the 87th Precinct*. New York: Random House, 1994. ISBN: 0688102212

Mitcham, Judson. *The Sweet Everlasting*. Atlanta: University of Georgia Press, 1996. ISBN: 0820318078

Palahniuk, Chuck. *Choke: a Novel*. New York: Doubleday, 2001. ISBN: 0385501560

Parker, Gary E. *The Wedding Dress*. Colorado Springs, CO: Cook Communications Ministries, 2002. ISBN: 0781437008

Raney, Deborah. *A Vow to Cherish*. Minneapolis: Bethany House, 1996. ISBN: 155661666X

Rogge, Robert H. *The Rat's Tale: Alzheimer's Mystery Story*. Chapel Hill, NC: Longleaf Press, 1997. ISBN: 0965731901

Rushford, Patricia H. *Now I Lay Me Down to Sleep*. Minneapolis, MN: Bethany House, 1997. ISBN: 1556617305

Sabatini, Sandra. *The One with the News*. Erin, ON: Porcupine's Quill, 2000. ISBN: 0889842175

Siddons, Anne Rivers. *Fault Lines*. New York, NY: Harper & Collins, 1995. ISBN: 0060176148

Smith, Martin J. *Shadow Image*. New York: Jove Books, 1998. ISBN: 0515122866

Sparks, Nicholas. *The Notebook*. New York: Warner Books, 1999. ISBN: 0446676098

Szeman, Sherri. *Only with the Heart: a Novel*. New York: Arcade Pub., 2000. ISBN: 1559705388

Tem, Melanie. *The Tides*. New York: Leisure Books, 1996. ISBN: 0843945745

Trocheck, Kathy Hogan. *Lickety-Split: a Truman Kicklighter Mystery*. New York: Harper & Collins, 1996. ISBN: 0060176415

Turner, George. *The Destiny Makers*. New York: Morrow, 1993. ISBN: 068812187X

Wiesel, Elie. *The Forgotten*. Translated by Stephen Becker. New York: Summit Books, 1992.

Williams, S. L. *A Secret Journal.* 1st Books, 2001. ISBN: 0759615799

Wright, Camron Steve. *Letters for Emily: a Novel.* New York: Pocket Books, 2001. ISBN: 0743444469

5

Books for Children and Teenagers

Altman, Linda Jacobs. *Alzheimer's Disease*. San Diego, CA: Lucent Books, 2001. ISBN: 1560066954

Altman, Linda Jacobs. *Singing with Mama Lou*. New York: Lee & Low Books, 2002. ISBN: 158430040X

Bahr, Mary. *The Memory Box*. Morton Grove, IL: A. Whitman, 1992. ISBN: 0807550523

Ballmann, Swanee. *The Stranger I Call Grandma: a Story about Alzheimer's Disease*. St. Cloud, FL: Jawbone Publishing, 2001. ISBN: 0970295944

Bauer, Marian Dane. *A Dream of Queens and Castles*. New York, NY: Clarion Books, 1990. ISBN 0395513308.

Bauer, Marion Dane. *An Early Winter*. New York: Clarion Books, 1999. ISBN: 0395903726

Beckelman, Laurie. *The Facts about Alzheimer's Disease*. New York: Crestwood House, 1990. ISBN: 0896864898

Bracken, Rosemarie. *Keeping Memories Alive*. Abingdon, MD: Memory Lane Press (P. O. Box 284, Abingdon, MD 21009)

Brown, Marian Tally. *Grandma Has Alzheimer's But It's OK*. 1stBooks Library, 2001. ISBN: 0759622213

Casey, Barbara. *Grandma Jock & Christabelle.* Nashville, TN: James C. Winston Pub. Co., 1995. ISBN: 1555234062

Check, William A. *Alzheimer's Disease.* New York: Chelsea House, 1989. ISBN: 0791000567 (hardback); 079100483X (paperback)

Evans, Eileen. *It's Me Grandma! It's Me!* Bridgeport: Alzheimer Disease Society; Sloane & Partner, Weymouth, 1992. ISBN: 0951832905.

Frank, Julie. *Alzheimer's Disease: the Silent Epidemic.* Minneapolis, MN: Lerner Publications, 1985. ISBN: 0822515784

Gold, Susan Dudley. *Allie Learns about Alzheimer's Disease: a Family Story about Love, Patience, and Acceptance.* (Special Family and Friends Series.) Plainview, NY: JayJo Books, 2001. ISBN: 1891383159

Gold, Susan Dudley. *Alzheimer's Disease.* Enslow Publishers, 2000. Rev. ed. (Health Watch Series.) ISBN: 0766016501

Graber, Richard. *Doc.* New York: Harper & Row, 1986. ISBN: 0060220643; 0060220945 (library binding)

Groot, Tracy. *The Mystery of the Forgotten Fortune.* Wheaton, IL: Crossway, 1996. (Casey and the Classifieds; bk. 2.) ISBN: 0891079114

Gruenewald, Nancy. *Grandpa Forgot My Name.* Austin, MN: Newborn Books, 1997. (Newborn Books, 508 South Main Street, Austin, MN 55912).

Guthrie, Donna. *Grandpa Doesn't Know It's Me.* New York: Human Sciences Press, 1986. ISBN: 0898853087.

Harmon, Daniel E. *Life Out of Focus: Alzheimer's Disease and Related Disorders.* Philadelphia: Chelsea House Publishers, 1999. ISBN: 0791048969

Hinnefeld, Joyce. *Everything You Need to Know When Someone You Love Has Alzheimer's Disease.* Portland, OR: Multnomah, 1989. ISBN: 082391688X

Karkowsky, Nancy Faye. *Grandma's Soup*. Rockville, MD: Kar-Ban Copies, 1989. ISBN: 0930494989 (hardback); 0930494997 (paperback)

Kehret, Peg. *Night of Fear*. New York: Minstrel Book, Published by Pocket Books, 1994. ISBN: 0671892177

Kelley, Barbara. *Harpo's Horrible Secret*. Prairie Grove, AR: Ozark Pub., 1996. ISBN: 1567630588 (hardback); 1567630596 (paperback)

Kibbey, Marsha. *My Grammy*. Minneapolis, MN: Carolrhoda Books, 1988. ISBN: 0876143281

Klein, Norma. *Going Backwards*. New York: Scholastic, 1986. ISBN: 0590403281 (hardback); 05940329X (paperback)

Kroll, Virginia L. *Fireflies, Peach Pies, & Lullabies*. New York: Simon & Schuster, 1995. ISBN: 0027510018

Laminack, Lester L. *The Sunsets of Miss Olivia Wiggins*. Atlanta: Peachtree Publishers, 1998. ISBN: 1567451398 (See Chapter 10, Reviews of Selected Books.)

Landau, Elaine. *Alzheimer's Disease*. New York: Franklin Watts, 1996. ISBN: 0531112683

Langdon, Mary Janine. *When Meme Came to Live at My House*. M. J. Langdon; New York: Printed by Phoenix Home Life Mutual Insurance Co, 1997. ISBN: 0967168805

Leavey, Peggy Dymond. *Help Wanted, Wednesday's Only*. Toronto: Napoleon Publishing, 1994. ISBN 0929141237

Leighton, Audrey O. *A Window of Time*. Lake Forest, CA: NADJA, 1995. ISBN: 0963633511

Mackall, Dandi Daley. *Horse Whispers in the Air*. St. Louis, MO: Concordia Pub. House, 2000. ISBN: 0570070082

Mahy, Margaret. *Memory*. New York: Alladin Paperbacks, 1997. ISBN: 0689829116

Marvis, B. *Coping with Alzheimer's Disease*. Chelsea House, 1996. ISBN: 0791043533

Nelson, Micheaux Vaunda. *Always Gramma*. New York: G. P. Putnam's Sons, 1988. ISBN 0399215425.

Park, Barbara. *The Graduation of Jake Moon*. New York: Atheneum Books for Young Readers, 2000. ISBN: 068983912X

Potaracke, Rochelle. *Nanny's Special Gift*. New York: Paulist Press, 1994. ISBN: 0809166151

Rappaport, Doreen. *But She's Still My Grandma*. New York, NY: Human Sciences Press, 1982. ISBN 089885072X

Sakai, Kimiko. *Sachio Means Happiness*. San Francisco: Children's Book Press, 1990. ISBN: 0892390654

Sanford, Doris. *Maria's Grandma Gets Mixed Up*. Portland, OR: Multnomah, 1989. ISBN: 0880702982

Schein, J. *Forget-Me-Not*. Toronto: Annick Press, 1988. ISBN 1550370006 (paperback); 1550370014 (hardback)

Schwartz, Noa. *Old Timers: the One that Got Away!* Downsview, ON: Tumbleweed Press, 1998. ISBN: 0968330312 (paperback)

Shawyer, Margaret. *What's Wrong with Grandma?: a Family Experience with Alzheimer's*. Amherst, NY: Prometheus Books, 1996. ISBN: 1573921076

Shecter, Ben. *Great-Uncle Alfred Forgets*. New York: HarperCollins, 1996. ISBN: 0060262184; 0060262192 (library binding)

Smith, Doris Buchanan. *Remember the Red-Shouldered Hawk*. New York: G. P. Putnam's Sons, 1994. ISBN: 0399224432

Swallow, Pamela Curtis. *It Only Looks Easy*. Brookfield, CT: Roaring Brook Press, 2003. ISBN: 0761317902

Swinwood, Laurie. *Rainbows & Other Promises*. New Canaan Publishing Co., 1999. ISBN: 188965812X

Tall, Martin. *Popsicle Sticks*. San Jose: Writer's Club Press / iUniverse, 2002. ISBN: ISBN: 0595225187

Tonkin, Rachel. *Grandpa's Stories*. Port Melbourne, Victoria: Roland Harvey Books, 1996. ISBN: 0949714445

Walker-Blondell, Becky. *In My Mother's Arms*. Nashville, TN: Scythe Publications, 1995. ISBN: 0155523647

Weitzman, Elizabeth. *Let's Talk about When Someone You Love Has Alzheimer's*. New York: Rosen / PowerKids Press, 1996. ISBN: 0823923061

Whitelaw, Nancy. *A Beautiful Pearl*. Morton Grove, IL: A. Whitman, 1991. ISBN: 0807505994

Wild, Margaret. *Remember Me*. Albert Whitmore & Co., 1995. ISBN: 0807569348.

Wilkinson, Beth. *Coping When a Grandparent Has Alzheimer's Disease*. New York: Rosen Pub. Group, 1995. ISBN: 0823914151

Willett, Edward. *Alzheimer's Disease*. Enslow Publishers, 2002 (Diseases and People Series.) ISBN: 0766015963

Williams, Carol Lynch. *If I Forget, You Remember*. New York: Delacorte Press, 1998. ISBN: 0385325347

Willner-Pardo, Gina. *Figuring out Frances*. New York: Clarion Books, 1999. ISBN: 0395915104

Woodbury, Mary. *Jess and the Runaway Grandpa*. Regina: Coteau Books, 1997. ISBN: 1550501135

About the Elderly, Nursing Homes, Death, and Grief

Alley, R. W. *Sad Isn't Bad: a Good-Grief Guidebook for Kids Dealing with Loss.* Abbey Press, 1998. ISBN: 0870293214

Auch, Mary Jane. *Cry Uncle!* New York: Holiday House, 1987. ISBN: 0823406601

Bunting, Eve. *Sunshine Home.* New York: Clarion, 1994. ISBN: 0395633095

Carlstrom, Nancy White. *Blow Me a Kiss, Miss Lilly.* New York: Harper & Row, 1990. ISBN: 0060210125

Delton, Judy. *My Grandma's in a Nursing Home.* Albert Whitman & Company, 1986. ISBN 0807553336.

Dugan, Barbara. *Loop the Loop.* New York: Greenwillow Books, 1992. ISBN: 0688096476

Heegaard, Marge E. *When Someone Very Special Dies: Children Can Learn to Cope with Grief.* Woodland Press, 1992. ISBN: 0962050202

Kibbev, Marsha. *The Helping Place.* Minneapolis: Carolrhoda Books, 1991. ISBN: 0876146809

Munsch, Robert. *Love You Forever.* Willowdale, ON: Firefly Books, 1993. ISBN: 0920668364; 0920668372 (paperback) (See Chapter 10, Reviews of Selected Books.)

6

Alzheimer's and Caregiving Periodicals

Activities Directors' Quarterly for Alzheimer's and Other Dementia Patients. Weston, MA: Prime National Pub. Corp. Quarterly.

Advances: Progress in Alzheimer Research and Care. Chicago, IL: Alzheimer's Association. Quarterly.

Advice and Consent. P. O. Box 850, Lake Placid, FL 33852.

Alzheimer Advocate. Denver, CO: Alzheimer's Disease and Related Disorders Association, Metro Denver Chapter. Bimonthly.

Alzheimer Disease and Associated Disorders. Lawrence, KS: Western Geriatric Research Institute. Quarterly.

Alzheimer Insight. Bellingham, WA: Alzheimer's Society of Washington. Quarterly.

Alzheimer's Aid Society of Northern California Newsletter. Sacramento, CA: The Society.

Alzheimer's Association: Marin County Chapter Newsletter. San Rafael, CA: Marin Alzheimer's Association. Bimonthly.

Alzheimer's Association Metro Denver Chapter News. Denver, CO: Alzheimer's Association, Metro Denver Chapter. Bimonthly.

Alzheimer's Association National Newsletter. Alzheimer's Association, 919 North Michigan Ave. Suite 1000, Chicago, IL 60611-1676. Quarterly URL: *http://www.alz.org/*

Alzheimer's Association Newsletter. Baton Rouge, LA: Alzheimer's Association, Greater Baton Rouge Chapter. Bimonthly.

Alzheimer's Association Newsletter. Miami, FL: Alzheimer's Association, Greater Miami Chapter. Quarterly

Alzheimer's Book and Care Connections Newsletter. Betty Gibbs / Gibbs Associates, P. O. Box 706, Boulder, CO 80306-0706.

Alzheimer's Care Quarterly: ACQ. Frederick, MD: Aspen Publishers. Quarterly.

The Alzheimer's Caregiver. Houston, TX: Living Centers of American for Families and Friends.

Alzheimer's Disease and Associated Disorders. Hagerstown, MD: Lippincott, Williams & Wilkins URL: *http://www.alzheimerjournal.com/*

Alzheimer's Disease and Related Disorders Helpline Newsletter. Topeka, KS: Kansas Department on Aging.

Alzheimer's Disease Review. Lexington, KY: Sanders-Brown Center on Aging, University of Kentucky URL: *http://www.mc.uky.edu/adreview/*

Alzheimer's Home Companion. Reno, NV (P. O. Box 3577): Eymann Publications. URL: *http://www.care4elders.com/*

Alzheimer's Reports. Cambridge, UK: MSJ. Bimonthly.

Alzheimer's Research. Oxford, UK: New York: Rapid Science Publishers. Bimonthly.

Alzheimer's Research Review. Rockville, MD (15825 Shady Grove Road, Suite 140, Rockville, MD 20850): Alzheimer's Disease Research.

Alzheimer's Researcher News. Dallas, TX: The Center.

American Journal of Alzheimer's Care and Research. Weston, MA: Prime National Pub. Corp. Bimonthly.

American Journal of Alzheimer's Disease. Weston, MA: Prime National Pub. Corp., Bimonthly.

Answers: the Magazine for Adult Children of Aging Parents. P. O. Box 9889, Birmingham, AL 35220-0889.

The Caregiver. Durham, NC: Duke Alzheimer's Family Support Program. Quarterly.

Caregiving Newsletter. Tad Publishing Co., 114 Euclid, Ste. 270, Park Ridge, IL 60068 URL: *http://www.caregiving.com/*

Companion. Indianapolis, IN: Alzheimer's Association of Central Indiana. Bimonthly.

Connections: News from the ADEAR Center. Silver Spring, MD: The Center.

Day by Day: Caring for Patients with Alzheimer's Disease. Alzheimer's Family Care, a service of Parke-Davis, 630 9th Ave. Suite 901, New York, NY 10036.

Dementia and Geriatric Cognitive Disorders. S. Karger AG. URL: *http://www.karger.ch/journals/dem/dem%5Fjh.htm*

High Notes. Los Angeles: John Douglas French Foundation for Alzheimer's Disease.

Issues in Focus. Cleveland, OH: Alzheimer's Association Chapter. Quarterly.

Journal of Alzheimer's Disease. Amsterdam; Washington: IOS Press. Bimonthly.

National Newsletter. Toronto: Education Committee, Société Alzheimer Society. Quarterly.

Newsletter. Cleveland, OH: Alzheimer's Association Chapter. Quarterly.

Newsletter. Winnipeg: Alzheimer Society of Manitoba.

The Newsletter of the Alzheimer's Association from the Wyoming Chapter. Casper, WY: Alzheimer's Disease and Related Disorders Association. Quarterly.

Newsletter: the National Newsletter of the Alzheimer's Society. London: Alzheimer's Society.

Northern Nevada Newsletter. Reno, NV: Alzheimer's Association, Northern Nevada Chapter. Quarterly.

Outlook. Columbus, OH: Alzheimer's Association of Central Ohio.

Prairie View. Regina: Alzheimer Society of Saskatchewan. Quarterly.

Progress Report on Alzheimer's Disease. Bethesda, MD: U.S. Dept. of Health and Human Services, Public Health Service, National Institutes of Health, National Institute on Aging. Annual.

Reflects: the Newsletter of the Alzheimer Society of Manitoba. Winnipeg: Alzheimer Society of Manitoba. Bimonthly.

Report of the Advisory Panel on Alzheimer's Disease. Washington, DC: U.S. Dept. of Health and Human Services. Annual.

Research and Practice. Chicago, IL: Medical and Scientific Affairs Division of the Alzheimer's Association.

Research and Practice in Alzheimer's Disease. Paris: New York: Serdi Publisher; Springer Pub. Co. Annual.

Respite Report. Winston-Salem, NC: Bowman Gray School of Medicine, Dementia Care and Respite Services Program.

Sandwich Generation. Dept. W Box 132, Wickatunk, NJ 07765-0132 URL: *http://www.thesandwichgeneration.com/*

Southwestern Researcher: Newsletter of the Alzheimer's Disease Research Center. Dallas, TX: The Center.

Stand By News. Milwaukee, WI: Alzheimer's Association of Southeastern Wisconsin. Quarterly.

Support, Advocacy and Research News. Vancouver, BC: Alzheimer's Support Organization of British Columbia.

The Support Network News. Naples Florida Alzheimer's Support Network, 660 Tamiami Trail North, Suite 21, Naples, FL 34102 URL: *http://gator.naples.net/presents/Alzheimer/nwstoc.html*

Take Care!: Self-care for the Family Caregiver. Silver Spring, MD: National Family Caregivers Association. Quarterly.

Texas Alzheimer's News. Austin, TX: Texas Dept. of Health, Office of Special Projects. Quarterly.

Today's Caregiver Magazine. P. O. Box 800616, Miami, FL URL: *http://www.caregiver.com/*

The WAITC Connection. Milwaukee, WI: Wisconsin Alzheimer's Information and Training Center.

Wiser Now. Better Directions. P. O. Box 35, Spencerville, MD 20868.

Wyoming AlzHelper. Newcastle, WY: Wyoming Alzheimer's Association. Quarterly.

7

Filmography:
Alzheimer's and Caregiving
Videos

Alone...But Not Forgotten. Presented by the Alzheimer's Association. Durham, NC: Educational Media Services, Duke University Medical Center; Washington, DC: District of Columbia Office on Aging, 2000. (48 min.)

Alzheimer's 101: the Basis for Caregiving. South Carolina Commision on Aging; South Carolina Educational Television, 1994. (85 min.)

Alzheimer's: a Practical Guide for Sitters. Produced by Dementia Education and Training Program. Montgomery, AL: Dept. of Mental Health and Mental Retardation, 1995. 2 videocassettes. (28 min.) URL: *http://www. alzbrain.org/resource/videos.html*

Alzheimer's: a Practical Guide to Community Resources. Produced by Dementia Education and Training Program. Montgomery, AL: Dept. of Mental Health & Mental Retardation, 1994. (60 min.) URL: *http://www. alzbrain.org/resource/videos.html*

Alzheimer's: a Practical Guide to Pastoral Care. Produced by Dementia Education and Training Program. Tuscaloosa, AL: University of Alabama Center for Public Education, 1995. 2 videocassettes. (52 min.) URL: *http://www.alzbrain.org/resource/videos.html*

Alzheimer's Disease. Berch Stelly, Glen Mire, Rita Earl. Broadcast as an episode of House Calls 12/97; taped off-air from KADN-TV Channel 15, Lafayette, LA: Produced at K62TV Studio in conjunction with Our Lady of Lourdes Regional Medical Center; Lafayette, LA: KADN-TV; Our Lady of Lourdes Regional Medical Center, 1997. (30 min.)

Alzheimer's Disease. Christine York, Claude Desrosiers, Kelly Ricard. Evanston, IL: Altschul Group Corp., 1996. (14 min.)

Alzheimer's Disease. Dr. Machlan. Toronto: IMS Creative Communications, University of Toronto, 1988. (10 min.)

Alzheimer's Disease. Jamie Guth. Lebanon, NH: Dartmouth-Hitchcock Medical Center, 1997 (The Doctor is In Series.) (28 min.) URL: *http://www. dartmouth.edu/~drisin/videos/alz.shtml*

Alzheimer's Disease. Jerry Romig. Austin Summers. New Orleans, LA: Hotel Dieu Hospital, 1991. (30 min.)

Alzheimer's Disease. Kate Jackson, Peter Keefe. Seattle, WA: Unapix Entertainment; Trouble in Mind Productions, 1999. (50 min.)

Alzheimer's Disease. Laura Smith McKenna. St. Louis, MO: Mosby-Year Book, 1997. ISBN: 0815185758

Alzheimer's Disease: a Delicate Balance. Metro Toronto Community Services Dept. Toronto: Metro Toronto Community Services Dept., Homes for the Aged Division, 1990. (20 min.)

Alzheimer's Disease - a Wilderness Explored. Kenneth L. Davis. Research Triangle Park, NC: Glaxo Wellcome, 1997. (32 min.)

Alzheimer's Disease and Other Dementias. Mark Julian Campbell, Director.

Alzheimer Disease and the Family: the Real Victims. Toronto: Metro Homes for the Aged, 1988.

Alzheimer's Disease: at Time of Diagnosis. Everett Koop, Medical Director; Mike Schneider, Host. New York: Time Life Medical, 1996. (30 min.) ISBN: 1575770016. Contents: Understanding the diagnosis - What happens next? - Treatment & management - Issues & answers.

Alzheimer's Disease: Capturing Precious Moments. Barbara Jean Copeman-High. Carrollton, TX: PRIMEDIA Workplace Learning, 2002. (30 min)

Alzheimer's Disease: Care at Home. Toronto: Alzheimer Society of Canada, Home Support Canada, Frameworks Communications, 1993. (18 min.)

Alzheimer's Disease: Coping with Confusion. M. Gray-Vickery. Los Angeles: Hospital Satellite Network, 1985. (29 min.)

Alzheimer Disease Do's and Don'ts. Peter V. Rabins, Susan Hannah Hadary, W. A. Whiteford. Baltimore, MD: Video Press, 2000. (26 min.)

Alzheimer's Disease Family Education Videotape Series. Des Moines: Iowa Department of Elder Affairs, 1987. 4 videocassettes (127 min.) Contents: 1. The stages of Alzheimer's disease: implications for the family - 2. Financial and legal issues for family caregivers - 3. Caring for the caregiver: strategies for stress and guilt management - 4. Dependent adult abuse: responsibilities and avenues for assistance.

Alzheimer's Disease: Inside Looking Out. Cleveland, OH: Alzheimer's Association Cleveland Area Chapter, 1995. (18 min.)

Alzheimer's Disease: Is Today's Science Tomorrow's Management? Howard A. Crystal, Peter Davies. Secaucus, NJ: Network for Continuing Medical Education, 1991. (48 min.)

Alzheimer's Disease: Living in the Here and Now. Frank Field. Eisai Inc. and Pfizer Inc., 1999. (14 min.)

Alzheimer's Disease: Managing the Later Stages in the Home. Washington, DC: Veteran's Administration, 1989. (15 min.)

Alzheimer's Disease: Minimizing Care Problems. Peter V. Rabins. Baltimore, MD: Video Press, University of Maryland, School of Medicine, 1997. (20 min.)

Alzheimer's Disease: One Question at a Time, One Day at a Time. Brenda McDonough. Pfizer Inc. and Eisai Inc, 1997. (18 min.)

Alzheimer's Disease: Pieces of the Puzzle. James Robert Allender. Tucson, AZ: The University of Arizona, 1990. (2 hr.)

Alzheimer Disease: Responsive Care Plans. Peter V. Rabins. Baltimore, MD: Video Press, University of Maryland, School of Medicine, 1997. (20 min.)

Alzheimer's Disease: Stolen Tomorrows. Van Nuys, CA: AIMS Media, 1988. (26 min.)

Alzheimer's Disease: the Family Conference. Washington, DC: Veteran's Administration; Bedford, MA: Geriatric Research Education Clinical Center, 1989. (19 min.)

Alzheimer's Disease: the Journey Within. Arlo Grafton and S. Grafton, Sue Martin. (View from the inside series) Omaha, NE: Envision Communications, 1995. (20 min.)

Alzheimer's Disease: the Long Nightmare. Princeton, NJ: Films for the Humanities and Sciences, 1987. (19 min.)

Alzheimer's Disease: What Caregivers Need to Know. Tampa, FL: University of South Florida Suncoast Gerontology Center, 2000. (22 min.)

Alzheimer's Disease: You Are Not Alone. Park Ridge, IL: Retirement Research Foundation, 1984. (28 min.)

Alzheimer's: Effects on Patients and Their Families. Princeton, NJ: Films for the Humanities and Sciences, 1991. (19 min.)

Alzheimer's: Feeding and Dental Hygiene. J. Robert Boggs. Winona Lake, IN: Boggs Books, 1990. (37 min.)

The Alzheimer's Journey. Ontario: Alzheimer Society of Canada, 1998. 3 videos (16-18 min.) Contents: Module 1. The Road Ahead - Module 2. On the Road - Module 3. At the Crossroads.

The Alzheimer's Mystery. Laurence Serfaty. Princeton, NJ: Films for the Humanities & Sciences, 2000. (48 min.)

Alzheimer's: No Easy Answers. Toronto: Metro Homes for the Aged, 1988.

An Alzheimer's Story. New York: Filmakers Library, 1985. (28 min.)

Alzheimer's: the Tangled Mind. Princeton, NJ: Films for the Humanities & Sciences, 1998. (26 min.)

Amanda's Choice. Canadian Broadcasting Corporation. New York: Filmakers Library, 2001. (48 min.)

Another Home for Mom. Lori Hope. Boston: Fanlight Productions, 1991. (28 min.)

Best Friends. Michael Lombardi. Baltimore, MD: Alzheimer's Association, Lexington/Bluegrass Chapter, Helping Hand Program. Distributed by Health Professions Press, 1997. ISBN: 1878812386 (15 min.)

The Best They Can Be: Communicating with People who Have Alzheimer Disease. Toronto: Metro Homes for the Aged, 1988.

Bringing Out the Best. (Dementia Programming and Activities series) Winston-Salem, NC: Partners in Caregiving, The Dementia Services Program, Bowman Gray School of Medicine of Wake Forest University, Department of Psychiatry and Behavioral Medicine, 1994. 4 videocassettes (ca. 356 min.) Contents: Tape 1. Direct care techniques (part 1) - Tape 2. Direct care techniques (part 2) - Tape 3. Activity ideas and resources - Tape 4. Administrative concerns.

Bubblegum, Buttermilk, & Leprechauns. Michelee Puppets. Orlando, FL: Alzheimer Resource Center, 1995. (19 min.)

Caregiver Issues. Linda Teri, James Lurie, Linda Keatley. Seattle, WA: University of Washington, Alzheimer's Disease Research Center, 1990. (33 min.)

The Caregiver's Dilemma: Detecting Treatable Medical Problems in the Alzheimer Patient. Kenneth Brummel-Smith. California: The Media Services, 1986. (45 min.)

Caregiving with Grace. Susan Hadary Cohen and W.A. Whitford. Baltimore: Video Services, 1987.

Caring about Howard. Durham, NC: Duke University, 1997. (23 min.)

Caring…Families Coping with Alzheimer's Disease. Chicago, IL: Alzheimer's Disease and Related Disorders Association, 1985. (28 min.)

Caring for Residents with Alzheimer's Disease. Global Village Communications Productions. Dayton, OH: Miami Valley Alzheimer's Association Chapter, 1993. (20 min.)

Caring for the Caregiver. Chicago: Alzheimer's Association, 1990. (20 min.)

Clinical Profiles in Alzheimer's Disease: Mild, Moderate and Severe. Pfizer Inc and Eisai Co., 1998. (25 min.)

Comfort for Alzheimer's Families. Bethlehem, PA: Robin Miller, Filmaker URL: *http://www.filmaker.com/videos.htm*

Communicating with Moderately Confused Older Adults. Duluth, MN: Mental Health Outreach Network, 1997. (20 min.)

Communicating with Severely Confused Older Adults. Duluth, MN: Mental Health Outreach Network, 1997. (20 min.)

Communicating with the "Alzheimer-type" Population: the Validation Method. Edward R. Feil, Naomi Feil. New York: Filmakers Library, 1991. (21 min.) Contents: Marge, the blamer - Muriel the wanderer.

Communication Strategies for Alzheimer's Patients. Ruth M. Tappan. University of Miami School of Nursing. R. Tappan, 1987. (30 min.)

Compassionate Touch: Benefits and Effects in Alzheimer's Care. Dawn Nelson. Allen Touch Associates, 1995. (27 min.)

Complaints of a Dutiful Daughter. Deborah Hoffmann. New York: Women Make Movies, 1994. (44 min.)

The Confused Resident: Strategies for Quality Care. Edward G. McMahon, Judith B. Eighmy, Gail D. Azain, Nancy Hunter-Sheiner, Carol J Farran. Garden Grove, CA: Medcom/Trainex, 1990. (30 min.)

Coping with Aged Parents. Linda Reid, T. Franklin Williams, Carter Catlett Williams. Los Angeles, CA: Hospital Satellite Network, 1984. (58 min.)

Creating Moments of Joy. Jolene Brackey. Polk City, IA: Enhanced Living, 1999. ISBN: 1878812653 (1 hr. 47 min.). Contents: Understanding the person with Alzheimer's - Powerful tools that create positive outcomes - Memory enhanced environments.

The Crucible of Alzheimer's Disease: Moral, Ethical, and Emotional Issues. University of Southern California. Los Angeles: Biomedical Instructional Media Services, 1986. (58 min.)

Dancing Inside: an Alzheimer's Story. Auguste Productions, 1997.

Dealing with Alzheimer's Disease: a Common Sense Approach to Communication. Producer, Karen Feldt; Writer/Field Producer, Kermit Cantwell. St. Paul: Ramsey Foundation, 1990. (21 min.)

Dealing with Alzheimer's: Facing Difficult Decisions. Karen Feldt. St. Paul, MN: Chicago, IL: Ramsey Foundation; Distributed by Terra Nova Films, 1992. (20 min.)

Dealing with Problem Mealtime Behavior in Alzheimer's Residents. Barbara Haley, RN BSN. Tana Hinson Durnbaugh. Waukegan, IL: Lake County Health Department, 1993. (18 min.)

Dementia & Alzheimer's Caregiving: through the Looking Glass. Coastal Healthtrain. Virginia Beach, VA: Coastal Training Technologies Corp, 2002. (20 min.)

The Diary of Rozie Mock. Henry Stephen Vogel. Eugene, OR: Showplace, 1990. (28 min)

Do you remember love? Los Angeles: Fries & Distribution, 1985. (28 min.)

Early Onset Memory Loss: a Conversation with Letty Tennis. Produced by Joseph and Kathleen Bryan Alzheimer's Disease Center, Duke University Medical Center. Chicago: Terra Nova Films, 1992. (20 min.)

The Educated Caregiver Series. Nashville: Life View Resources 3 videos (2 hr. 58 min.). Contents: v. 1. Coping Skills - v. 2. Hands-on Skills - v. 3. Essential Knowledge. URL: *http://www.lifeviewresources.com/tec.htm*

Enhancing the Communication Ability of Alzheimer's Patients. Faerella Boczko. Vero Beach, FL: Speech Bin, 1997. (25 min.)

Facing Legal and Financial Considerations. Linda Haskins, Producer and Director. Urbana, IL: Carle Medical Communications, 1991. (21 min.)

A Family's Journey after Alzheimer's Diagnosis. Barbara Jean Copeman-High. Carrollton, TX: PRIMEDIA Workplace Learning, 2002. (30 min.)

Favorite Things. Marilyn Snell, Dale A. Lund. KUED-TV, University of Utah, Alzheimer's Association. Salt Lake City: Innovative Caregiving Resources, 1993. (33 min.)

Flowers for Peggy. Franklin K. Cassel. Lancaster, PA (Brethren Village, 3001 Lititz Pike): F. Cassel, 1997.

Forget Me Never. Based on the book, *Living in the Labryinth*, by Diana Friel McGowin. Mia Farrow, Martin Sheen; Directed by Robert Ackerman. Storyline Productions, Screen Adventures II, 1999.

From Here to Hope: the Stages of Alzheimer's Disease: Final, Middle, and Early. Duke University. Medical Center. Educational Media Services. Durham, NC: Duke University, 1998. (1 hr. 17 min.) Contents: Segment One. Final stage Alzheimer's disease - Segment Two. Middle stage Alzheimer's disease - Segment Three. Early stage Alzheimer's disease.

Front-row Seat: a Sing-a-long Video for Older Seniors and Alzheimer's Patients. Custom Video Productions / Novato. ISBN: 0967082404

Front-row Seat: More Oldies: a Sing-a-long Video for Older Seniors and Alzheimer's Patients. Directed by Barbara Jacobs. Custom Video Productions / Novato. ISBN: 0967082420

Front-row Seat: Sing-a-long with Barbara Songs for the Holiday Season. Directed by Barbara Jacobs. Custom Video Productions / Novato. ISBN: 0967082412

Glass Curtain. Doris Chase, Jennie Ventriss. White Plains, NY: Lucerne Media; Distributed by Terra Nova Films, 1983. (28 min.)

Glenn's Perspective on Grace. Glenn Kirkland, Grace Kirkland. Baltimore, MD: Video Press, University of Maryland at Baltimore, 1990. (20 min.)

The Goodbye. Vancouver, BC: Tideline Productions. (23 min.)

Grace. Susan Hadary Cohen and W.A. Whiteford. Participants Glenn Kirkland, Grace Kirkland. Baltimore, MD: Video Services, Dept. of Physical Therapy, School of Medicine, University of Maryland at Baltimore, 1990. (58 min.).

Grandpa Doesn't Know It's Me. Derry, NH: Chip Taylor Communications, 1995. (Donna Guthrie series.) (10 min.)

Home Care for People with Alzheimer's Disease. Produced by Vince Clews and Associates, Inc. Gaithersburg, MD: Aspen Publications, 1995. 3 videos (50 min.) ISBN: 0834207184 Contents: 1. Communication - 2. Activities of daily living - 3. Home safety.

Home is Where I Remember Things. Duke Aging Center. Duke University Durham, NC: Educational Media Services, Duke University Medical Center, 1998. (47 min.)

How to Communicate with Someone Who Has Alzheimer's Disease or Related Dementia. Written and directed by Marion Karpinski. Healing Arts Communications, 2001. (30 min.) ISBN: 0970555628

Impaired Communication. Peter V. Rabins. Baltimore: Video Press, 1993. (17 min.)

Improving Caregiving Skills. Susie Thurgood. Los Angeles, CA: Silver Spring, MD: University of Southern California, Alzheimer's Disease Center; Distributed by Alzheimer's Disease Education and Referral Center, 1991. (1 hr. 13 min.)

Improving the Ability of Alzheimer's Patients to Communicate. Kathryn A. Bayles, Cheryl K. Tomoeda. Tucson, AZ: Canyonlands Pub., 1998. (28 min.)

In and Out of Time. Elizabeth Finlayson. Hohokus, NJ: New Day Films, 1996. (14 min.) URL: *http://www.newday.com/films/In_and_Out_of_Time.html*

Interacting with Alzheimer Patients: Tips for Families and Friends. Peter V. Rabins. Baltimore, MD: Video Press, University of Maryland School of Medicine, 2000. (27 min.)

Interacting with Alzheimer's Patients: Tips for Family and Friends: Recognizing Caregiver Burnout. Peter V. Rabins. Baltimore, MD: Video Press, University of Maryland School of Medicine, 2000. (20 min.)

Just for the Summer. Alzheimer's Association, Los Angeles Chapter. Churchill Films, 1988. (30 min.)

Last List. Marilyn Holt, Carolyn Wood, Kathryn Atwood. Salt Lake City, UT: KUED, 1999. (60 min.)

Living in a Nightmare: a Public Affairs Presentation. Southfield, MI: WXYZ-TV, 1982. (30 min.)

Living in Alzheimer's Disease. George G. Glenner Alzheimer's Family Centers. San Diego: Office of Learning Resources, 1999. (60 min.)

Living with Alzheimer Disease: the Family Caregiver's Guide: Caregivers' Options. Peter V. Rabins. Baltimore, MD: Video Press, 1998. (20 min.)

Living with Alzheimer Disease: the Family Caregiver's Guide: Endings. Peter V. Rabins. Baltimore, MD: Video Press, 1998. (24 min.)

Living with Alzheimer Disease: the Family Caregiver's Guide: Ethical Issues. Peter V. Rabins. Baltimore, MD: Video Press, 1998. (21 min.)

Living with Alzheimer Disease: the Family Caregiver's Guide: The Beginning. Peter V. Rabins. Baltimore, MD: Video Press, 1998. (20 min.)

Living with Alzheimer Disease: the Family Caregiver's Guide: the Middle Years. Peter V. Rabins. Baltimore, MD: Video Press, 1998. (21 min.)

Living with Alzheimer Disease: the Family Caregiver's Guide: the New Relationship. Peter V. Rabins. Baltimore, MD: Video Press, 1998. (20 min.)

Living with Alzheimer's: a Partnership in Caring. Rochester, NY: Alzheimer's Association, Rochester NY Chapter; Chicago, IL: Distributed by Terra Nova Films, 1990. (19 min.)

Living with Grace. Baltimore, MD: Video Services, Dept. of Physical Therapy, School of Medicine, University of Maryland at Baltimore, 1983. (28 min.)

Losing it all, the Reality of Alzheimer's Disease. Producer, Writer, Director Michael Mierendorf. Princess Yasmin Aga Khan, Michael Mierendorf. (HBO Project Knowledge Series.) New York: HBO Studio Productions: Distributed by Ambrose Video Publishing, 1991. (54 min.)

Lost in the Mind: the Mystery of Alzheimer's Disease. Washington, DC: Don Lennox Productions, 1996. (90 min.)

Managing and Understanding Behavior Problems in Alzheimer's Disease and Related Disorders: the ABCs of Behavior Management in Dementia. Linda Teri, James Lurie. Seattle, WA: University of Washington, 1990. 10 videos (1 hr. 12 min.) Contents: 1. Overview. Part I, Alzheimer's disease and related diseases - 2. Overview. Part II, Delirium and depression - 3. ABCs, an introduction - 4. Managing aggressive behaviors, anger and irritation, catastrophic reactions - 5. Managing psychotic behaviors, language deficits - 6. Managing psychotic behaviors, hallucinations / delusions and paranoia and suspiciousness - 7. Managing personal hygiene, bathing and dressing - 8. Managing difficult behaviors, wandering and inappropriate sexual behaviors - 9. Managing difficult behaviors, depression - 10. Caregiver issues.

Managing with Alzheimer's Disease. Timonium, MD: Milner-Fenwick, 1983. (29 min.).

The Many Faces of Alzheimer Disease. Toronto: Alzheimer Society for Metropolitan Toronto, 1996. (14 min.)

Memories of Love: Caring for the Caregiver. University of Pittsburgh. Pittsburgh, PA: University of Pittsburgh. Alzheimer's Disease Research Center, 1993. (16 min.)

Memory, a presentation of Films for the Humanities & Sciences; Dana Alliance for Brain Initiatives; WETA. Barry Gordon, et al. Princeton, NJ: Films for the Humanities & Sciences, 1999. (57 min.)

My Challenge with Alzheimer's Disease. Beverly Wheeler. Philogenesis Productions. Chicago: Terra Nova Films, 1996. (16 min.)

My Promise to You: the Story of Robertson and Muriel McQuilkin. Grand Rapids, MI: Produced by RBC Ministries, 1999. (27 min.)

Not Alone in the World: Caring for Someone with Alzheimer's. Schoolhouse Videos. (22 min.)

The Other Victim: Coping & Caring Techniques for the Caregivers of Alzheimer's Patients. Dick Bakkerud. Chapel Hill, NC: Health Sciences Consortium, 1987. (48 min.)

A Part of Daily Life: Alzheimer's Caregivers Simplify Activities and the Home. Anne Morris. Bethesda, MD: American Occupational Therapy Foundation, 1993. ISBN: 1569000093 (17 min.)

A Partial View: an Alzheimer's Journal. Cary Henderson. Presented by the University of Virginia Medical School. Charlottesville, VA: University of Virginia Clinical Engineering Media Production Services, 1999. (60 min.)

Participating in Research: a Legacy of Hope. Alzheimer's Disease Education & Referral Center (National Institute on Aging); Northwestern University (Evanston, IL). Silver Spring, MD: Distributed by Alzheimer's Disease Education & Referral Center, 2000. (13 min.)

Poppy's Head. Australia: Angell Productions (130 Brooklyn Road, Brooklyn, NSW, Australia 2083), 1998. (23 min.) Age 12-16. AFI Award (Australian Film Institute), 1998.

Recognizing and Preventing Caregiver Burnout. Peter V. Rabins, Susan Hannah Hadary, W.A. Whiteford, University of Maryland, School of Medicine. Baltimore: Video Press, 2000. (24 min.)

The Road to Galveston. Michael Toshiyuki Uno, Cicely Tyson, Piper Laurie, Tess Harper. Hollywood, CA: Paramount Pictures, 1996. ISBN: 0792140850

Saving Memories: Enhancing Lives. Chicago: Alzheimer's Association; Glendale Heights, IL: Distributor, TV Access, 1999. (16 min.)

Signs & Symptoms of Alzheimer Disease. Peter V. Rabins. Baltimore, MD: Video Press, University of Maryland, School of Medicine, 1997. (20 min.)

The Silent Epidemic. New York: Filmakers Library, 1982. (26 min.)

Solving Bathing Problems in Persons with Alzheimer's Disease and Related Dementias. Philip D. Sloane, Ann Louise J. Barrick, Vanessa Honn. Chicago, IL: Alzheimer's Association, 1996. (22 min.)

Someone I Love has Alzheimer's Disease. Host-Narrator Shelley Fabares, Producer-Director Nancy Fernandez Mills; Produced for the Alzheimer's Association of Eastern MA. Newton, MA: Lifecycle Productions, 1993. (17 min.)

Someone I Once Knew. Paula S. Apsell; Timothy Johnson. Northbrook, IL: MTI Teleprograms, 1983. (30 min.)

Something Should Be Done about Grandma Ruthie. Cary Stauffacher. Boston, MA: Fanlight Productions, 1993. ISBN: 1572951222 (54 min.)

Sonia. Paule Baillargeon. Ottawa: National Film Board of Canada, 1987. (54 min.)

Surviving Dementia. Pathway Productions. (38 min.)

There Were Times, Dear: about Living with Alzheimer's Disease. Shirley Jones. Los Angeles, CA: Direct Cinema Limited, 1986. (60 min.).

A Thousand Tomorrows: Intimacy, Sexuality, and Alzheimer's. Daniel Kuhn, James Vanden Bosch. Chicago: Distributed by Terra Nova Films, 1995. (32 min.)

Timeslips: Creative Storytelling with People with Dementia. Chicago: Terra Nova Films, 1998. (10 min.)

To Care: a Portrait of Three Older Caregivers. Boston, MA: Consumers Union, 1987. (28 min.) ISBN: 1572951737

Understanding Alzheimer's Disease. Pittsburgh, PA: University of Pittsburgh, 1993. (31 min.)

Understanding the Communication Problems of Alzheimer's Patients. Kathryn A. Bayles, Cheryl K. Tomoeda. Tucson, AZ: Canyonlands Pub., 1998. (35 min.)

Voices of Caregiving: Insights along The Way. Senior Video Project, Medicare Alzheimer's Project, Terra Nova Films. Chicago, IL: Terra Nova Films, 1994. (32 min)

A Vow to Cherish. Based on the book by Deborah Raney. Barbara Babcock, Ken Howard, Ossie Davis, John Schmidt. Minneapolis: World Wide Pictures Home Video, 1999. (1 hr. 12 min.)

Waves of Stone. Vision Associates; Glaxo. Vision Associates, 1994. (57 min.)

When Someone You Love Has Alzheimer's: A Practical Guide for Caregivers. Bill R. Irwin. Timonium, MD: Milner-Fenwick; Medcom, 1995. (32 min.)

When the Mind Fails. Princeton, NJ: Films for the Humanities & Sciences, 2000. (58 min.)

Whispering Hope: Unmasking the Mystery of Alzheimer's. New York: FBC Productions (136 East 57th St., New York, NY 10022. Phone: (212) 838-6268), 1984. (52 min.)

You Must Remember This: Inside Alzheimer's Disease. New York, NY: Filmakers Library, 1992. (57 min.).

Audiocassettes

Alzheimer's Disease, Religion, and Spirituality. Cleveland, OH: Fairhill Center for Aging, Alzheimer's Association, Cleveland Area Chapter, 1998. 7 audio-cassettes.

Bayly, John. *Elegy for Iris.* Read by David Case. Books on Tape, 1999. ISBN: 0736644725

Caregiver. Chicago, IL: Alzheimer's Association, 1990 (50 min.) Caregiving at home - Especially for the Alzheimer caregiver - Communicating with the Alzheimer's patient - Alzheimer disease: caring for the caregiver by Mike Fitzgerald.

Champion, Eric. *Glimpses of Grace: a Family Struggles with Alzheimer's.* Living History Press, 1998. ISBN: 096480462X

Communicating with Alzheimer's Patients. Rockville, MD: American Speech-Language-Hearing Association, 1999. 2 sound cassettes.

DeBaggio, Thomas. *Losing My Mind: an Intimate Look at Life with Alzheimer's.* Narrated by Cotter Smith. Simon & Schuster Audio, 2002. ISBN: 0743521099

Every Day's a Great Day. Alzheimer's Association North Bay Chapter, 1997.

Gass, Kathleen Ann. *The Alzheimer's Patient.* Madison, WI: Continuing Education in Nursing, 1986. (45 min.)

Gass, Kathleen Ann. *The Caregiver of the Alzheimer's Patient.* Madison, WI: Continuing Education in Nursing, 1986. (54 min.)

McGowin, Diana Friel. *Living in the Labryinth: a Personal Journey through the Maze of Alzheimer's.* Thorndike, ME: Thorndike Press, 1994. ISBN: 0786299762

Park, Barbara. *The Graduation of Jake Moon*. Narrated by Fred Savage. Listening Library, 2000. ISBN: 0807261602

Steps for Caregivers: Caring for Persons with Alzheimer's Disease. Produced by the Alzheimer's Association. Chicago, IL: Alzheimer's Association, 1998. (48 min.)

8

Books about Other Related Dementias

Huntington's Disease

Archer, Elton. *Red the Rose, Sharp the Thorn.* Longview, TX: Hudson Printing & Graphic Design, 1995.

Fosburgh, Liza. *The Wrong Way Home.* New York: Bantam Books, 1990. ISBN: 0553058835 [juvenile fiction]

Funk, Carrie L. *One Family's Experience with Genetic Testing for Huntington's Disease.* Columbus, OH: Ohio State University, 2000.

Guthrie, Marjorie. *A Family Member Speaks about Huntington's Disease.* New York: Huntington's Disease Society of America, 1979.

Jones, Randi. *Walking the Tightrope: Living at Risk for Huntington's Disease.* New York: Huntington's Disease Society of America, 1996. ISBN: 1963773011

Karlen, Richard R. *Devil's Dance.* Ironbound Press, 1998. ISBN: 0966083105

Kraus, Harry L. *Could I Have This Dance?* [a novel] Grand Rapids: Zondervan, 2002. ISBN: 0310240891

Leal-Pock, Carmen. *Faces of Huntington's*. Belleville, ON: Essence Publishing, 1998. ISBN: 1894169107

Leal-Pock, Carmen. *Portraits of Huntington's*. Belleville, ON: Essence Publishing, 2001. ISBN: 1553062515

Leonard, Alison. *Tina's Chance*. New York: Penguin Putnam Books for Young Readers, 1992. ISBN: 0140328823 [juvenile fiction]

Paulson, Jane S. *Understanding Behavior in Huntington's Disease: a Practical Guide for Individuals, Families and Professionals Coping with HD*. New York: Huntington's Disease Society of America, 1999. ISBN: 1963773046

Phillips, Dennis H. *Living with Huntington's Disease: a Book for Patients and Families*. Madison, WI: University of Wisconsin Press, 1992. ISBN: 0299086704

Pollard, Jim. *A Caregiver's Handbook for Advanced Stage Alzheimer's Disease*. New York: Huntington's Disease Society of America, 1999. ISBN: 0963773038

Quarrel, Oliver. *Huntington's Disease: the Facts*. New York: Oxford University Press, 1999. ISBN: 0192629301

Rubalcaba, Jill. *St. Vitus' Dance*. New York: Clarion Books; Houghton-Mifflin, 1996. ISBN: 0395727685. [juvenile fiction]

Stevens, David Lawrence. *Huntington's Chorea: a Booklet for the Families and Friends of Patients with the Disease*. London: Association to Combat Huntington's Chorea, 1975.

Understanding Huntington's Disease: a Resource for Families. Cambridge, ON: Huntington Society of Canada, 1995.

Werbel, Eileen. *Toward a Fuller Life: a Guide to Everyday Living with Huntington's Disease*. New York, NY: Huntington's Disease Society of America, 1990.

Wexler, Alice. *Mapping Fate: a Memoir of Family, Risk, and Genetic Research.* New York: Times Books; Random House, 1995. ISBN: 0812917103

Pick's Disease

The Official Patient's Sourcebook on Pick's Disease: a Revised and Updated Directory for the Internet Age. ICON Group International, 2002. ISBN: 0597829993

Strokes/Vascular Dementia/Multi-Infarct Dementia

Ashman, Shirley. *Living Daily with Dementia: "It Wasn't Me".* Bishop Auckland: Pentland, 2001. ISBN: 1858219493

Bosworth, Kathy. *Your Mother Has Suffered a Slight Stroke.* America House Book Publishers, 1992. ISBN: 1588512886

Hay, Jennifer. *Stroke: Questions You Have - Answers You Need.* People's Medical Society, 1995. ISBN: 1882606221

Hodges, Houston. *Circle of Years: a Caregiver's Journal.* Morehouse Publishing, 1998. ISBN: 0819217484

Meyer, John Stirling. *Vascular Dementia.* Mount Kisco, NY: Futura Pub., 2001. ISBN: 0879934255

Senelick, Richard C. *Living with Stroke: a Guide for Families - Help and Hope for All Those Touched by Stroke.* New York: McGraw-Hill Contemporary, 1999. ISBN: 0809226073

9

Books About Grief and Loss

Akner, Lois F. *How to Survive the Loss of a Parent: a Guide for Adults.* New York: Morrow, 1993.

Bowlby, J. *Attachment and Loss, v. III, Loss.* New York: Basic Books, 1980.

Bozarth, Alla Renee. *A Journey through Grief: Gentle, Specific Help to Get You Through the Most Difficult Stages of Grieving.* Hazelden Information & Educational Services, 1990. ISBN: 1568380372

Bradley, June S. *Walk in My Shoes: Living with Grief.* San Jose: Writer's Club Press / iUniverse, 2001. ISBN: 0595201385

Browne, Sylvia. *A Journal of Love and Healing: Transcending Grief.* Hay House, 2001. ISBN: 1402847823

Bullitt, Dorothy. *Filling the Void: Six Steps from Loss to Fulfillment.* New York: Rawson Associates, 1996.

Dawson, Ann. *A Season of Grief: a Comforting Companion for Difficult Days.* Ave Maria Press, 2002. ISBN: 0877939780

Donnelly, Katherine Fair. *Recovering from the Loss of a Parent.* San Jose: iUniverse, 2001. ISBN: 0595140378

Figley, C.R. *Trauma and Its Work.* New York: Bruner / Mozel, 1985.

Fitzgerald, Helen. *The Mourning Handbook: a Complete Guide for the Bereaved*. New York: Simon & Schuster, 1994.

Grief Therapy. Edited by Karen Katafiasz. Abbey Press, 1993. ISBN: 0870292676

Herman, J. *Trauma and Recovery*. New York: Basic Books / Harper-Collins, 1992.

Hickman, Martha Whitmore. *Healing After Loss: Daily Meditations for Working through Grief*. William Morrow, 1994. ISBN: 0380773384

Johnson, Margaret E. *Beyond Heartache: Comfort & Hope for Hurting People*. San Jose: Author's Choice Press / iUniverse, 2000. ISBN: 0595010768

Koman, Aleta. *How to Mend a Broken Heart: Letting Go and Moving On*. Chicago: Contemporary Books, 1997.

Kushner, H.S. *When Bad Things Happen to Good People*. New York: Schocken Books, 1981.

Letters from Motherless Daughters: Words of Courage, Grief and Healing. Edited by Hope Edelman. Dell, 1996. ISBN: 0385315228

Levy, Alexander. *The Orphaned Adult: Understanding and Coping with Grief and Change after the Death of Our Parents*. Perseus Publishing, 2000. ISBN: 0738203610

Lewis, C.S. *A Grief Observed*. New York: Simon & Schuster, 1986.

McCarthy, Sherri. *A Death in the Family: a Self-help Guide to Coping with Grief*. Vancouver: Self-Counsel Press, 1988.

Manning, Doug. *Don't Take My Grief Away from Me*. In-Sight Books, 1980. ISBN: 1892785048

Manning, Doug. *Share My Lonesome Valley: the Slow Grief of Long-Term Care*. In-Sight Books, 1999. ISBN: 1892785331

Martin, John D. *I Can't Stop Crying: It's So Hard When Someone You Love Dies*. Toronto: Key Porter Books Limited, 1992.

Menten, Theodore. *After Goodbye: How to Begin Again after the Death of Someone You Love*. Philadelphia: Running Press, 1994.

Menten, Theodore. *Gentle Closings: How to Say Goodbye to Someone You Love*. Philadelphia: Running Press, 1991.

Moody, Raymond A. *Life after Loss: Conquering Grief and Finding Hope*. San Francisco: Harper, 2001. ISBN: 0062517295

Moore, James W. *When Grief Breaks Your Heart*. Nashville: Abingdon Press, 1995. ISBN: 0687007917

Rando, Therese A. *Grieving: How To Go On Living When Someone You Love Dies*. Lexington, MA: Lexington Books, 1988.

Raphael, B. *The Anatomy of Bereavement*. New York: Basic Books, 1984.

Roberts, Barbara K. *Death Without Denial, Grief Without Apology: a Guide for Facing Death and Loss*. New Sage Press, 2002. ISBN: 0939165430

Stearns, A. *Living through Personal Crisis*. Chicago: Thomas More Press, 1984.

Tansley, Tangea. *For Women Who Grieve: Embracing Life after the Death of Your Partner*. Freedom, CA: The Crossing Press, 1996.

Tatelbaum, J. *The Courage to Grieve: Creative Living, Recovery & Growth through Grief*. New York: Harper-Collins.

Temes, Roberta. *Living with an Empty Chair: a Guide through Grief*. Roberta Temes. New York: Irvington Publishers, 1983.

Westberg, Granger E. *Good Grief: a Constructive Approach to the Problem of Loss*. Augsburg Fortress Pub., 1983. ISBN: 0800611144

Wolfelt, Alan D. *Understanding Grief: Helping Yourself Heal*. Taylor and Francis, 1992. ISBN: 1559590386

Zimmerman, Susan. *Writing to Heal the Soul: Transforming Grief and Loss through Writing*. Crown Publishers, 2002. ISBN: 060980829X

Zonnebelt-Smeenge, Susan J. *Getting to the Other Side of Grief: Overcoming the Loss of a Spouse*. Grand Rapids: Baker Books, 1998. ISBN: 080105821X

10

Reviews of Selected Books

The 36-Hour Day, by Nancy L. Mace and Peter V. Rabins. Baltimore: Johns Hopkins University, 1991.

This is the most recommended book about Alzheimer's disease. It is required reading for every caregiver. The first Alzheimer's Association chapter I contacted sent me a copy of it the first time I called them, and for that I will always be grateful. Not until I had read this book did I better understand Alzheimer's and what it was doing to my mother. Read every book you can find on Alzheimer's, but you will probably want to read this one first.

Alzheimer's Disease: Caregivers Speak Out, by Pam Haisman. Fort Myers, FL: Chippendale House Publishers, 1998.

Pam Haisman is a nurse consultant for Alzheimer's disease who went on the Internet to gather the stories of caregivers. Her book tells the facts about Alzheimer's, the statistics, and about the research that is being done, but the bulk of the book is the stories of caregivers, as the cover tells: "In their own words families seek compassion, professionals relate frustrations, spouses share their grief, teenagers pledge their love". This book expresses the emotions of caregiving as no other book has in allowing over 200 caregivers to speak out about what it is really like.

Elder Rage: or, Take My Father…Please! How To Survive Caring for Aging Parents, by Jacqueline Marcell. Irvine, CA: Impressive Press, 2001.

In this highly acclaimed book, Jacqueline Marcell tells her caregiving story, of her raging dementia patient father, of her sweet feeble mother, and of her "Amazing Ariana", the caregiver who helped her through it all. Jacqueline gave up a career as a television executive to care for her parents, but she didn't give up adventure - as we who have been caregivers know, there are surprises every-day around Alzheimer's/dementia patients. Jacqueline also has an Internet radio show called "Coping with Caregiving", and I have been one of the hon-ored guests. As she interviewed me, I felt such a kinship with Jacqueline having shared similar experiences, the same emotions of frustration, guilt, and grief, and now, the same mission - helping others to avoid the mistakes we made in caregiving. Show archives URL: *http://www.ElderRage.com/ShowArchive.asp*

Faces of Huntington's, by Carmen Leal-Pock. Belleville, ON: Essence Publishing, 1998.

Although this book is not about Alzheimer's it is about a related dementia. Carmen is caregiver for her husband, who has Huntington's Disease, the dis-ease which my ex-husband's mother had. On her Web site and in support groups both off and online, Carmen gathered the stories, poems, and thoughts of many affected by this hereditary disease. She included a poem I wrote about my ex-mother-in-law, "Growing Old Fast", and a couple others from my Web site, because as she has said on her site, "Though the name of the diseases are different, many of the symptoms, caregiving challenges, and emotions are the same". This book gives us a lot of insight into the challenges and emotions of those affected by this disease, about which little was known until the past few years. Carmen has done a wonderful job in raising an aware-ness of this disease through her Web site and this book.

Failure-Free Activities for the Alzheimer's Patient, by Carmel Sheridan. Forest Knolls, CA: Elder Books, 1995.

"What kind of activities are there for the Alzheimer's patient?" is a question that comes up often on the Alzheimer list, and one that I am asked pretty often. I always recommend this book. Carmel describes all kind of activities:

music, exercise, food preparation, crafts, gardening, solo activities, family games, and reminiscence. I especially like the chapter on reminiscence, featuring the life collage, memory book, memory box, and more. Activities are very important, as is explained in this book's introduction: "The more involved patients remain with the world around them, the more resourceful they become at finding ways to keep that world from slipping away."

Finding the Words: A Communication Guide for those who Care, by Harriet Hodgson Minneapolis, MN: John Wiley, 1995.

"Finding the words" to communicate with someone who has Alzheimer's is a problem, especially after many words have lost their meanings to that person. Harriet Hodgson, the daughter of an Alzheimer's patient, has done an excellent job in giving us a guidebook for communicating in the daily struggle all caregivers go through, as she gives us many anecdotes from her personal experience with her mother. In this book we learn about communication at all stages of the disease, the causes of communication problems, and how to "run interference" or how to identify and deal with "the obstacles before they deal with us." We can't fix things; we can't make everything right for the person with Alzheimer's, but we can try to achieve better communication, realizing as the author says in her epilogue: "It isn't easy for caregivers to find the words they want. Some days we succeed; other days we fall short of our goal. The important thing is that we're trying to improve communication. And that we keep on trying because we care."

Gone Without a Trace, by Marianne Dickerman Caldwell. Forest Knolls, CA: Elder Books, 1995.

Imagine your mother wandering off from a school softball game. Imagine searching frantically for her for three years. Imagine her remains being found in the woods where she had died. This happened to Marianne Dickerman Caldwell's mother. Stella Mallory Dickerman was an educated woman who had gone back to get her Master's degree after having her children. She was a teacher, an artist, and a world-traveler. She also had Alzheimer's disease. At age

83, on a September day in 1991, Stella went for a walk, and she was never seen again. Marianne Caldwell's book about this experience is not only a very poignant and personal story, but it also offers comfort and guidance to families who have experienced loss and assistance for families who are searching for a missing loved one. Marianne gives a sample query letter, missing persons profile, and letter to a medical examiner. She also lists the addresses and phone numbers for the Alzheimer's Association's Safe Return Program and for State Agencies on Aging, as well as other helpful organizations. Marianne is also the Director of the Home Safely Foundation and is the creator of Birthnet for Wanderers which is a free I.D. registry system for the dementia patient.

Grandpa Forgot My Name, by Nancy Gruenewald; illustrated by Bruce Loeschen. Austin, MN: Newborn Books, 1997. (Newborn Books, 508 South Main Street, Austin, MN 55912)

In this wonderful children's book by Nancy Gruenwald, Grandpa came to live with the family because he couldn't take care of himself anymore. Dad helped him dress and mom helped him eat his vegetables, but Grandpa doesn't forget how to eat cookies and doughnuts... and ice cream. This delightful book is based on the author's family experiences with a grandpa who lived with them for a year before he died. Its message is clear, that caregiving is a rewarding experience though not an easy one, and though the grandpa in the story forgot his grandaughter's name, he didn't forget he loved her.

He Used to Be Somebody: a Journey into Alzheimer's Disease through the Eyes of a Caregiver, by Beverly Bigtree Murphy. Boulder, CO: Gibbs Associates, 1995.

In a 348 page book that reads like a novel, Beverly Bigtree Murphy tells a love story of a lifetime of love shared in a few years with her husband, Tom Murphy, as he began his descent into Alzheimer's disease. Soon after their whirlwind romance culminated in marriage, Tom's successful career began to decline as the disease they would later come to know as Alzheimer's began its destruction of his brilliant mind and charismatic personality. Beverly soon found herself thrust into the role of caregiver for her beloved new husband,

and into legal battles concerning his care, as well as going in circles in search of medical help before the diagnosis of Alzheimer's. The emotional turmoil caregivers know well is shared in Beverly's story, along with practical advice from her as a professional as well as a caregiver. Her book also includes the stages of Alzheimer's, an annotated list of books Beverly found most helpful, and other suggested reading on grief and positive thinking as well as Alzheimer's and caregiving. Beverly's Web site offers practical suggestions to help with incontinence care and for dealing with challenging behaviors as well as information about her book. *He Used to Be Somebody* is a story of unconditional love, a love that did not end even through all the turmoil brought about by Alzheimer's. The old love song lyrics at the beginning of each chapter are just one more evidence of this, weaving together the story of Tom and Beverly Murphy and their unending love. URL: *http://www.bigtreemurphy.com/*

Learning to Sit in Silence: a Journal of Caretaking, by Elaine Marcus Starkman. Watsonville, CA: Papier-Mache Press, 1993.

This book features short journal entries and poetry, spanning over three years when Elaine Starkman's life was consumed by taking care of her mother-in-law who had a dementia that was probably Alzheimer's. The first year she took care of her in her home, juggling her caretaking responsibilities with caring for a husband and teenage children. The next two years her mother-in-law was in a nursing home, but the stress was still there. The disease progressed so fast, especially after the nursing home entry. This book takes us from the early stages of dementia through the last stages and death. This is an enlightening book, and one which was helpful to me. I read it in March 1995 while I was taking care of my mother.

Living in the Labyrinth: a Personal Journey through the Maze of Alzheimer's, by Diana Friel McGowin. New York: Delacorte Press, 1993.

This amazing book is written by the Alzheimer's victim herself. Diana Friel McGowin began having symptoms of Alzheimer's disease at age 45. She gives us an inside look at what it is like to have this disease, from the first symptoms noticed, through the ordeal of searching for a diagnosis, to the finality in the diagnosis itself and the daily losses that come. Diana has a wonderful attitude, finding comfort in her memories of simple things: the smell of the small town library of her childhood, the taste of icicles on her tongue, the sight of the first daffodils of spring, lightning bugs, a train whistle, her grandmother's violin. What a wonderful way to view it all, as she says "I can sometimes enjoy the sweet fragrance of night blooming jasmine when no one else can." We, the children of Alzheimer's victims, hope that a cure can be found, but if it does-n't come in our time, we do have an example of radiant acceptance. *Living in the Labryinth* is also available in large print (published by Thorndike Books, P. O. Box 159, Thorndike, ME 04986) and in an audio-book version. It is a best seller and has been published in eleven languages.

Looking for Mother (a book of poetry) by Hugh MacDonald. ON: Black Moss Press, 1995. Distributed by Firefly Books, Ltd. (3680 Victoria Park Ave. Toronto, ON M2H 3K1) ISBN 0887532594; 0887532551

This book of poetry by award-winning poet and childrens' book author, Hugh MacDonald, is about his mother and Alzheimer's disease. Hugh takes us on the journey from cherished memories of childhood into the tragic world of his mother's Alzheimer's, yet we still sense the beauty that remained through it all. Several of Hugh's poems from this book are featured in *Alzheimer's Poetry* at *A Year to Remember*. *Looking for Mother* won the top prize in the 1994 Atlantic Poetry Competition. Hugh's book, *Chung Lee Loves Lobsters* won the L. M. Montgomery Childrens' Literature Award in 1990. He teaches English and History at a high school near Charlottetown, Prince Edward Island.

Love You Forever, by Robert Munsch. Willowdale, ON: Firefly Books, 1993.

"I'll love you forever, I'll like you for always, as long as I'm living my baby you'll be," was the song sung to the little boy in the story, even when he was two and had flushed his mother's watch down the toilet, even when he was nine and never wanted to take a bath, even when he was a teen and wore strange clothes and listened to strange music, even when he was grown up and lived across town. So when his mother was old and sick, the man returned her love, and he sung a similar song for her as he cared for her, and when she died he picked up his own baby and sung his mother's song of love to that child. A beautiful, touching book everyone of all ages should read. I read it just before I went home to be my mother's caregiver, and I cried so hard then; and I still cannot stop the tears each time I read it. Although not about Alzheimer's, it is certainly relevant to caregiving.

One Family's Journey through Alzheimer's Disease, by Mary B. Walsh. Wheaton, IL: Tyndale House, 2000.

Going through having a loved one with Alzheimer's is enough, but that's not all that happens to most of us during that time; there are many other family concerns, and so many stories to tell. Mary Walsh tells them all in this wonderful book that will make you laugh at times and cry at others. Mary's husband's grandmother and her Alzheimer's is the focus of this book, and it is around this that most of both the funny and tearful stories revolve. Mary and her family cared for "Gram" during the years I was with my mother as her caregiver. "Gram" died in a nursing home in May 1996, in the month following my mother's death, and there are many similarities. Unlike me, however, but probably like many of you, Mary had the concerns of four generations of family members who were surrounding her. If you are a caregiver or former caregiver of someone with Alzheimer's, I am sure that you, too, will find much in common with this family's story. Mary presents it delightfully in a very readable manner which includes conversation, journal entries, and her poems. Through all the tears and the laughter, the family's strong faith shines through, and if you are a caregiver, you will be encouraged through reading this book, and you will know that you, too, can make it.

Painted Diaries: A Mother and Daughter's Experience through Alzheimer's, by Kim Howes Zabbia. Minneapolis, MN: Fairview Press, 1996.

Covering a period of eleven years (1982-1993) in the life of one family, this touching book chronicles one woman's Alzheimer's journey through her own journal entries and the paintings and journal of her daughter, Kim. Among treasured family photos is a 1982 group picture of four generations, including Kim's mother, her grandmother, and her daughter at nine weeks old. There is even a photo of the mother's declining writing, as she wrote "I love you" in the fall of 1989. As the years passed and the disease progressed in her mother's life, Kim found her paintings influenced by the disease. Her paintings changed as she explored her family's emotional struggle and visualized her mother's feelings in her work. Kim and her mother's journey was aided by their creativity in helping them cope, understand, and express the changes brought about by what her mother called "Al, Mrs. Zheimer's son".

Passage into Paradise, by Dorothy Womack. San Jose: Writer's Club Press / iUniverse, 2002.

You may have enjoyed Dorothy Womack's poetry in her *Reflections* on Marsha Penington's *Alzheimer's Outreach*, at *A Window on My Mind*, and in *Alzheimer's Poetry* at *A Year to Remember*. Now available in book form, her experience as her mother's caregiver is shared in *Passage into Paradise*. I was amazed as I read her story, which began years before mine, and continued several months after my mother died. I do not think I could have handled caring for my mother as Dorothy and her husband did. Long after her mother became bedridden and incontinent, still they cared for her at home. Dorothy's honesty in this book, expressing all the emotional turmoil she was going through, combined with her strong faith shining through, make this a story we become caught up in. I found I just had to read it all at one sitting, and it is a story that I will want to read again and again.

The Reluctant Caregivers: Learning to Care for a Loved One with Alzheimer's, by Anne Hendershott. Westport, CT: Bergin & Garvey, 2000.

Anne Hendershott, a professor who teaches about the sociology of aging, found herself unprepared for the challenge of caring for a mother-in-law with Alzheimer's. Combining the personal experience of a caregiver, who had a family and career as well, with the knowledge of a professional, this book can be very helpful to others who reluctantly find themselves in the role of caregiver. Practical information and tips from lessons learned in that role are shared along with this personal caregiving journey. A helpful appendix includes facts about organizations and selected Web sites, and a bibliographic essay shares information about helpful books. I am honored and grateful to Anne Hendershott for including *A Year to Remember* among the recommended Web sites in the Appendix of *The Reluctant Caregivers*.

Show Me the Way to Go Home, by Larry Rose. Forest Knolls, CA: Elder Books, 1996.

This is another fascinating story actually written by an Alzheimer's patient in the early stages of the disease. Larry was diagnosed at age 54. This came after his getting lost on a trip, driving more than a hundred miles out of the way of the route to his destination before realizing it. Larry tries to see the good in this, writing that he has "more compassion for people, birds, deer, and the like" and he says "If when you read this book you feel a certain sadness…let yourself be sad, but not for me…I have had a good and prosperous life…Most of all, I have had the love of some beautiful people…and I have loved them, too."

This Stranger in Our House, by Jerry Ham. Spokane, WA: The Inland Northwest Chapter of the Alzheimer's Association (720 W. Boone Ave., Suite 101, Spokane, WA 99201), 1999.

Proclaimed the Poet Laureate of the *Alzheimer List* (Washington Univ. at St. Louis) by members of that support group and mailing list, Jerry Ham has stirred our emotions and caused us to shed healing tears as we have read his wonderful poems. This book includes "Yes I'll Cry" also posted in *Alzheimer's Poetry* at *A Year to Remember,* and thirteen other poems by Jerry, who is caregiver to his mother who has Alzheimer's disease. Published by his Alzheimer's Association Chapter in the state of Washington, all proceeds from the sale of his book (only $5.00 per copy) go to that Chapter. I am so proud that, other than on the *Alzheimer List,* my site was the first Web site, I think, where Jerry Ham's poems were posted. Other poems by Jerry at *Alzheimer's Poetry* are "She's Still My Mother", "My Dear I Love You", "A Prison of the Mind", and my very favorite one, which still brings tears every time I read it, "A Passing of Memory". If you would like to purchase a copy of Jerry's book, please e-mail Joel Loiacono at *joel.loiacono@alz.org* or call the Inland Northwest Chapter of the Alzheimer's Association at (509) 483-8456 or (800) 256-6659.

The Sunsets of Miss Olivia Wiggins, by Lester Laminack. Atlanta: Peachtree Publishers, 1998.

Miss Olivia just sits with her hands folded in her lap and stares, saying nothing. Her daughter Angel and great-grandson Troy visit, and she still sits as they talk to her. She still says nothing, but she thinks of beautiful memories from her past, beautiful as the sunset the nurse had pointed out that evening. Beautifully illustrated by Constance R. Bengum, this wonderful book was written by Lester Laminack, who went to the same high school as I. Though it was published in 1998, I did not discover this book until Christmas 2001 when I was visiting my sister and she showed me the copy she had purchased. It is such a beautiful book, and a wonderful gentle and loving story that can help young and old cherish their loved ones who have Alzheimer's.

Therapeutic Caregiving: a Practical Guide for Caregivers of Persons with Alzheimer's and Other Dementia Causing Diseases, by Barbara J. Bridges. Mill Creek, WA: BJB Publishing, 1995.

This book is indeed "a practical guide" for not only getting through each day, but also making each one better than it might have been otherwise. The chapters on communication and cueing will help in developing skills that will help make each day more pleasant, as will the chapters on preventing stress and managing problem behaviors. I was especially impressed with the "What If" questions in chapter seven, for example "What if you went to bed and didn't know whether it was nighttime or daytime? What if you woke up from a nap in the afternoon and thought it was time for breakfast? What if you became frightened or lost in a darkened room?" (p. 62) These questions help us to imagine what it is like for an Alzheimer's patient. All of this, plus the day-to-day eating, sleeping, hygiene, and even exercise is covered in this book by Barbara J. Bridges, a RN who spent fourteen years caring for both of her parents. I highly recommend this book for all caregivers URL: *http:// pages.prodigy.com/bjbservices*

To Hold a Falling Star: a Personal Story of Living at Home with Alzheimer's, by Betty Baker Spohr. Seattle: Longmeadow Press, 1990.

This is the story of a wife's eleven year journey with her husband through his Alzheimer's experience from the very early stages when he was diagnosed through three very difficult years when he became incontinent, almost immobile, and violent. The nursing home was an option that was always put off with "maybe I can go on a little longer", and then Betty's husband died of a heart attack. I read this book in March 1995, and I wrote this comment in a notebook: "This book makes me feel that I, too, can go on a little longer with things as they are. I just don't think I can put my mother in a nursing home - not yet, and this book inspires me with the kind of love it takes to hold on longer."

Conclusion

With more and more books being published, poems being written, and films being produced, it is difficult to conclude a book like this, and indeed, I could have worked forever on it, not feeling ever completely caught up. A book such as this one will in a sense be a bit incomplete and out of date as soon as it is published. Thus updating and revision will be a continuous process. I welcome additions, corrections, and suggestions, all of which may be submitted to me by e-mail at *bpsibley@mindspring.com* or mailed to me at P. O. Box 1625, Decatur, AL 35602-1625.

Best wishes, and may God bless Alzheimer's patients and caregivers everywhere!

About the Author

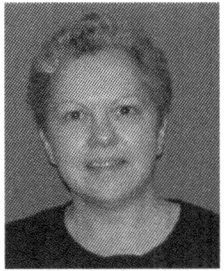

Brenda Parris Sibley's mother had Alzheimer's disease, and Brenda was her caregiver for sixteen months in 1994-1995. She died at age 80 after four months in a nursing home. Begun in 1996 in her mother's memory, Brenda's Web site, *A Year to Remember* (URL: *http://www.zarcrom.com.users/yeartorem/*) has grown to over 400 pages. Included are her caregiving journal, poetry, photos, links to Alzheimer's and caregiving resources, contributed poetry, stories and articles, and a bibliography and filmography.

Brenda had left graduate school needing twelve more semester hours when she moved in with her mother to be her caregiver. Although she was not able to go back at first, she did in January 1998, and graduated in December of that year. Brenda is Technical Services / Reference Librarian at Calhoun Community College in Decatur, Alabama. She is also the Library Webmaster.

Brenda's first book, *Waiting for the Morning: a Mother and Daughter's Journey through Alzheimer's Disease* was published by Writer's Club Press / iUniverse in 2001. It includes her poetry, caregiving journal, treasured family photos, and a brief bibliography and webliography.

Brenda is Contributing Editor for Suite101's Alzheimer's Topic at *http://www.suite101.com/welcome.cfm/alzheimers_disease* and she is also the list owner of *Top Alzheimer's/Caregiving Sites* at *http://new.topsitelists.com/bestsites/bpsibley/*.

Appendix A

Internet Resources

Webliography
Internet Informational Resources for Caregivers

Ageless Design: Smarter, Safer Living for Seniors - *http://www.agelessdesign.com/*

Agenet: Solutions for Better Aging - *http://agenet.agenet.com*

AlzBrain.org: Alabama's Alzheimer's Resource (Alabama Dementia Education and Training Program) - *http://www.alzbrain.org*

Alzheimer Europe - *http://www.alzheimer-europe.org/*

The Alzheimer Page (Washington University at St. Louis) - *http://www.adrc.wustl.edu/alzheimer/*

> The Alzheimer Mailing List - *http://www.adrc.wustl.edu/alzheimer/faq/faq.htm#subscribe*

> Alzheimer List Archives - *http://www.adrc.wustl.edu/hyperlists/alzheimer/*

Alzheimer's Association - *http://www.alz.org/*

> Find your local Alzheimer's Association Chapter - *http://www.alz.org/findchapter.asp*

Alzheimer's Directories at *Alzheimer Outreach -*
http://www.zarcrom.com/users/alzheimers/

Alzheimer's Disease Information Directory at *A Year to Remember -*
http://www.zarcrom.com/users/yeartorem/index4.html

Alzheimer's Support Network (Naples, Florida) -
http://home.sprintmail.com/~alznet/

Assisted Living Info - *http://www.assistedlivinginfo.com/*

The Care Guide: Canada's Premiere Guide to Senior Housing and Care Services -
http://www.assistedlivinginfo.com/

Caregiver.com/Today's Caregiver Magazine - *http://www.caregiver911.com/*

Caregiver Information - *http://caregiver-information.com/*

The Caregiver Network - *http://www.caregiver.on.ca/*

The Caregiver's Handbook - *http://www.acsu.buffalo.edu/~drstall/hndbk0.html*

The Caregivers (San Francisco Examiner Series) -
http://www.sfgate.com/examiner/caregivers/

The Caregiver's S.E.A.D: Support and Education for Alzheimer's Disease -
http://neuro-oas.mgh.harvard.edu/sea/

Caregiving.com - *http://www.caregiving.com/*

ElderCare Online - *http://www.ec-online.net/*

Eldercare Web - *http://www.elderweb.com/*

Empowering Caregivers - *http://www.care-givers.com/*

National Family Caregiver's Association - *http://www.nfcacares.org/*

Nursing Home Info - *http://www.nursinghomeinfo.com/*

The Ribbon Online - *http://www.theribbon.com/*

Signpost to Older People and Mental Health Matters Journal -
http://signpostjournal.connect-2.co.uk/

Suite 101 Alzheimer's Disease Topic -
http://www.suite101.com/welcome.cfm/alzheimers_disease

Virtual Law Office Alzheimer's Information -
http://www.virtuallawoffice.com/alz.html and Caregiver's Corner -
http://www.virtuallawoffice.com/investor.html

RESEARCH WEB SITES

Alzheimer's Disease Cooperative Study - *http://antimony.ucsd.edu/*

Alzheimer's Disease Research Center, Washington University at St. Louis - *http://alzheimer.wustl.edu/adrc2/*

American Association for Geriatric Psychiatry - *http://www.aagpgpa.org/*

Cognitive Neurology and Alzheimer's Disease Center, Northwestern University Medical School - *http://www.brain.nwu.edu/*

Dana Foundation/Dana Alliance for Brain Initiatives - *http://www.dana.org/*

Doctor's Guide to Alzheimer's Disease - *http://www.pslgroup.com/alzheimer.htm*

Geropsychology Central - *http://www.premier.net/~gero/geropsyc.html*

Joseph and Kathleen Bryan Alzheimer's Disease Research Center, Duke University Medical Center - *http://adrc.mc.duke.edu/*

Kingshill Research Center, Victoria Hospital, UK - *http://www.kingshill-research.org/*

Massachusetts Alzheimer's Disease Research Center - *http://neuro-www2.mgh.harvard.edu/adrc_home/*

Mayo Alzheimer's Disease Research Center, Mayo Clinic - *http://www.mayo.edu/research/alzheimers_center/*

National Institute of Neurological Disorders and Stroke - *http://www.ninds.nih.gov/*

Neurology at Massachusetts General Hospital - *http://neuro-www.mgh.harvard.edu/*

Neurosciences on the Internet - *http://www.neuroguide.com/*

Partners Program of Excellence in Alzheimer's and Other Neurogenerative Diseases - *http://neuro-oas.mgh.harvard.edu/alzheimers/*

Southern Illinois University Center for Alzheimer's Disease and Related Disorders - *http://www.siumed.edu/neuro/cadrd.html*

Suncoast Gerontology Center, University of South Florida - *http://www.med.usf.edu/suncoast/alzheimer/*

Stanford/VA Alzheimer's Research Center of California - *http://arcc.stanford.edu/*

UAB Alzheimer's Disease Center, University of Alabama at Birmingham - *http://main.uab.edu/show.asp?durki=11627*

University of Kansas Medical Center Alzheimer's Disease and Memory Disorders Clinic - *http://adc.kumc.edu/clinic/clinic.html*

The Whole Brain Atlas - *http://www.med.harvard.edu/AANLIB/home.html*

OTHER RELATED DEMENTIAS

Creutzfeldt-Jakob Disease

CJD Voice - *http://members.aol.com/larmstr853/cjdvoice/cjdvoice.htm*

Huntington's Disease

Huntington Society of Canada - *http://www.hsc-ca.org/*

Huntington's Disease Society of America - *http://www.hdsa.org/*

Lewy Body Disease

Lewy-Net - *http://www.nottingham.ac.uk/pathology/lewy/lewyhome.html*

Parkinson's Disease

AlzBrain.org on Parkinson's Disease - *http://www.alzbrain.org/misc/parkinsons.html*

Parkinson's Disease Society of Canada - *http://www.parkinson.ca/*

Parkinson's Society Canada -*http://www.parkinson.ca/home.html*

Pick's Disease

Pick's Disease Support Group - *http://www.pdsg.org.uk/*

Picks Information Page - *http://www.bhoffcomp.com/coping/picks.html*

Strokes/Vascular Dementia

AlzBrain.org on Vascular Dementia - *http://www.alzbrain.org/misc/vdementia.html*

National Stroke Association - *http://www.stroke.org/*

National Stroke Foundation, Australia - *http://www.strokefoundation.com.au/*

ONLINE SUPPORT DISCUSSION LISTS AND CHATS

The Alzheimer Mailing List -
http://www.adrc.wustl.edu/alzheimer/subscribe.html from the Alzheimer Page -
http://www.adrc.wustl.edu/alzheimer/, at Washington University of St. Louis,
including the list Archives - *http://www.adrc.wustl.edu/alzheimer/*

AD Book Reviews - *http://groups.yahoo.com/group/ADbkreviews/*

Adult Children of Dementia-Alzheimer's -
http://groups.yahoo.com/group/adult-children-of-dementia-alzheimers/

Advanced Alzheimer's - *http://groups.yahoo.com/group/advanced-alzheimer/*

After Alzheimer's Spouse -
http://groups.yahoo.com/group/AfterAlzheimersSpouse/

alt.support.alzheimers -
http://groups.google.com/groups?q=alt.support.alzheimers

alt.support.disabled-caregivers -
http://groups.google.com/groups?q=alt.support.disabled.caregivers

alt.support.grief - *http://groups.google.com/groups?q=alt.support.grief*

Alzheimer - *http://groups.yahoo.com/group/alzheimer/*

Alzheimer's - *http://groups.yahoo.com/group/alzheimers/*

Alzheimer's Care - *http://groups.yahoo.com/group/Alzheimerscare/*

Alzheimer's Caregivers - *http://groups.yahoo.com/group/AlzheimersCaregivers/*

Alzheimer's Circle of Friends -
http://groups.yahoo.com/group/Altzheimercircleoffriends/

Alzheimer's Club - *http://groups.yahoo.com/group/alzheimersclub/*

Alzheimer's Disease - htt*p://groups.yahoo.com/group/AlzheimerDisease/*

Alzheimer's Partners - *http://groups.yahoo.com/group/alzheimerspartners/*

Alzheimer's Related Dementia - *http://groups.yahoo.com/group/alzheimersrelateddementia/*

Alzheimer's Support - *http://groups.yahoo.com/group/alzheimerssupport/*

AlzHumor - *http://groups.yahoo.com/group/Alzhumour/*

AlzTalk - *http://groups.yahoo.com/group/AlzTalk/*

Caregiver's Army - *http://groups.yahoo.com/group/CAREGIVERSARMY/*

Carers - *http://groups.yahoo.com/group/carers/*

CWPML - Coping with Personal Memory Loss - *http://groups.yahoo.com/group/CWPML/*

DASN - Dementia Advocacy and Support Network - *http://groups.yahoo.com/group/DASN/*

DementiaSupport2 - *http://groups.yahoo.com/group/dementiasupport2/*

Dementia Teachers - *http://groups.yahoo.com/group/dementiateachers/*

Early Memory Loss - *http://groups.yahoo.com/group/earlymemoryloss/*

ElderCare Chat - *http://www.ec-online.net/Community/chatschedule.htm*

ElderCare Chat Guide - *http://groups.yahoo.com/group/ElderCareChatGuide/*

ElderCare Message Board - *http://216.122.139.136/cgi-bin/ultimatebb.cgi*

Friends Family of Alzheimer's - *http://groups.yahoo.com/group/friendsfamilyofalzheimers/*

Griefnet Mailing Lists/Support Groups - *http://rivendell.org/*

Kids Seeking Answers - *http://groups.yahoo.com/group/kidsseekinganswers/*

Loving Caregivers - *http://groups.yahoo.com/group/Loving_Caregivers/*

My Mother Has Alzheimer's -
http://groups.yahoo.com/group/mymotherhasalzheimers/

Neurology Web Forums - *http://neuro-www.mgh.harvard.edu/forum/*

Sons and Daughters - *http://groups.yahoo.com/group/sonsanddaughters2/*

Teen Caregivers - *http://groups.yahoo.com/group/TeenCaregivers/*

Teens Talking about Alzheimer's -
http://groups.yahoo.com/group/TeensTalkingAboutAlzheimers/

Top Alzheimer's/Caregiving Sites Newsletter -
http://groups.yahoo.com/group/TopADCaregivingSites/

YOD - Young Onset Dementia - *http://groups.yahoo.com/group/yod/*

PERSONAL WEB SITES BY CAREGIVERS, ALZHEIMER'S/DEMENTIA PATIENTS, AND PROFESSIONALS

Pages by Family Caregivers

Adult Caregivers - *http://home.earthlink.net/~sayitnow/caregiver.htm*

Alzheimer's Angels, by Dorothy Womack - *http://www.geocities.com/womack47/alzangels.html*

Alzheimer's Disease in Our Family, by Marilyn Sheaffer - *http://www.rain.org/~caspita/ad.html*

Alzheimer's Journey - *http://www.alzheimersjourney.com/*

Alzheimer's Outreach, by Marsha Penington - *http://www.zarcrom.com/users/alzheimers/index1.html*

Alzwell, by Susan Grossman/ElderCare Online - *http://www.webcom.com/~susan/welcome.html*

Blue Skies, by Dorothy Womack - *http://www.geocities.com/womack47/blueskies.html*

Bob Hoffman's Family Homepage - *http://www.bhoffcomp.com/coping/*

Carla's Page - *http://www.angelfire.com/ma/alrac/*

Coping with Alzheimer's Disease, by Denise Cooper - *http://www.geocities.com/HotSprings/3004/*
(Note: Denise passed away of lung cancer in 2002)

DORIED Alzheimer Pages - *http://www.geocities.com/Heartland/Pointe/3894/DAP/Alzheimer.htm*

Faith Walks On - *http://www.geocities.com/ibelieve1959/*

Grandmother Misty's Caregivers Site - *http://www.geocities.com/ladymisty2001/index.html*

Innerquest, by Dorothy Womack -
http://www.geocities.com/womack47/innerquest.html

Joanne Cares - *http://joanncares.homestead.com/homepage.html*

Joanne's Journal - *http://users.nac.net/jbsun/*

Kate's Place, by Katherine Murphy - *http://home.att.net/~katesdrm/*

LadyDove's Poems, by Carolyn Haynali -
http://www.ladydovespoems.homestead.com/LadyDove.html

LaVonne's Journey with Alzheimer's -
http://www.members.shaw.ca/traceylaird/main.html

Leave 'em Laughin' Darlin', by Brenda Race -
http://www.geocities.com/brace03/giggles.html

The Long Goodbye, by Penny Klein -
http://www.geocities.com/Wellesley/Garden/5337/

A Map for the Journey, by Sandra Cobb -
http://www.geocities.com/heartland/7015/alzheimr.html

Paintings by Vivian Hanby, by Dorothy Womack -
http://www.geocities.com/womack47/paintings.html

Passage into Paradise, by Dorothy Womack -
http://www.geocities.com/womack47/passage.html

Poems, Prayers, and Promises, by Brenda Race -
http://www.geocities.com/brace03/Mom.html

Sharon's Place Grandma's Page -
http://www.geocities.com/Heartland/Meadows/6396/gramma.html

Shekinah Glory, by Carolyn Haynali -
http://www.caregiversarmy.com/Carolyn/home.htm

Stella's Story - *http://www.geocities.com/stellasstory*

By People with Alzheimer's or a Related Dementia

Alice's Place, by Alice E. Young -
http://www.geocities.com/allieyoung1/Alices_Journals.html

Aloha, from Jeannie L. Lee in Hawaii, by Jeannie Lee -
http://www.angelfire.com/hi4/jleehawaii/

Alzheimer's Disease,Multiple Sclerosis & DID/MPD, by Laura Smith -
http://www.ycsi.net/users/laura/

Jan/Mina's Journey through Alzheimer's - *http://www.janmina.com*

Mary's Place, by Mary Lockhart -
http://www.angelfire.com/ok4/mari5113/

Morris Friedell's Home Page - *http://members.aol.com/MorrisFF/*

My Journey, by Chip Gerber -
http://www.zarcrom.com/users/alzheimers/chip.html

Simple Pleasures, by Peter Smith -
http://www.zarcrom.com/users/alzheimers/peter1.html

Teresa's Journal -
*http://pages.*ivillage.com/*resa526/alzheimers.html*

Thru His Eyes, by Tim Brennan -
http://www.nhisgarden.com/his_eyes/entrance.html

A Tribute to Arlene Francis - *http://www.arlenefrancis.com*

Memorials

All about My Grandpa, by Lisa -
http://www.angelfire.com/mi/fave/family.html

In Loving Memory of William M. Schutte, (father of Kim Schutte Holbrook, former Executive Director of the North Alabama Chapter of the Alzheimer's Association) - *http://www.kscon.com/bill.htm*

On Wings of Love: a Tribute to my Mother, by Fanny - *http://www.angelfire.com/pa2/fanny/tribute.html*

Undying Love, by Patrick Davidson - *http://denver.rockymountainnews.com/undyinglove*

A Year to Remember, by Brenda Parris Sibley - *http://www.zarcrom.com/users/yeartorem/*

Professionals' Homepages

BJB Geriatric Care Management, by Barbara J. Bridges - *http://pages.prodigy.net/bjbservices/*

Caregiver's Haven, by Nancy Walker - *http://www.nhisgarden.com/caregivers/entrance.html*

The Elderly Place, by Marci Stocks - *http://www.geocities.com/~elderly-place/*

Pam's Place on the Web - http://www.cp-tel.net/pamnorth/

ALZHEIMER'S AND THE ARTS ON THE INTERNET

Arts in Aging, from Huffington Center on Aging -
http://www.hcoa.org/arts/arts_in_aging_front.htm

Medical Humanities, from New York University School of Medicine -
http://endeavor.med.nyu.edu/lit-med/medhum.html

Art

ABC News.com Slideshow of Alzheimer's Patients' Art -
http://more.abcnews.go.com/sections/living/slides/alzheimers/

Heather Hill Hospital Residents' Artwork -
http://www.heatherhill.com/artsale.html

Jennifer Hiscox, Artist - http://www3.ns.sympatico.ca/yonder/website/Jframes.html

A Map for Moira - http://www.merseyworld.com/moira/

Memories in the Making at the Orange County California Chapter of the Alzheimer's
Association - *http://www.alz.org/chapters/template/orange/special.memmaking.1.htm*

"Memory, Spirit Stay Alive on Canvas at Alzheimer's Art Show" -
http://www.post-gazette.com/magazine/19981116art2.asp

The Painting of Vivian Hanby (mother of Dorothy Womack) -
http://www.zarcrom.com/users/yeartorem/paintings.html

Photo Gallery inspired by *A Window on My Mind*'s poetry -
http://neuro-mancer.mgh.harvard.edu/zeggeren/photography.html

Poetry

Alzheimer's and Aging: Poets Kelly Cherry and John Daniel write about
Alzheimer's - *http://www.wpr.org/book/segment%201*

Alzheimer's Outreach Poetry Gallery -
http://www.zarcrom.com/users/alzheimers/poetry.html

Alzheimer's Poetry, contributed poetry at *A Year to Remember* -
http://www.zarcrom.com/users/yeartorem/ADpoetry/contributed.html

Bibliography of Alzheimer's in Poetry, at *A Year to Remember* -
http://www.zarcrom.com/users/yeartorem/inpoetry.html

Other Literatures

Alzheimer's Bibliography for Children and Teenagers, at *A Year to Remember* -
http://www.zarcrom.com/users/yeartorem/AlzBibKids.html

Bibliography of Alzheimer's in Fiction, at *A Year to Remember* -
http://www.zarcrom.com/users/yeartorem/fiction.html

Film

Iris: New Miramax film about Iris Murdoch, author and Alzheimer's victim -
http://www.miramaxhighlights.com/iris/

GRIEF RESOURCES ONLINE

Bill Chadwick's Grief Resources Page - *http://www.premier.net/~zoom/*

Crisis, Grief, and Healing, by Tom Golden - *http://www.webhealing.com/*

Fernside Online: A Center for Grieving Children - *http://www.fernside.org/*

Griefnet.org - *http://rivendell.org/*

GrowthHouse.org on Grief and Bereavement - *http://www.growthhouse.org/death.html*

GROWW Grief Recovery - *http://www.groww.com/gr.htm*

Living with Grief: When a Loved One is Dying - http://www.caregivertips.com/helpful_links.htm

WidowNet - *http://www.widownet.org*

APPENDIX B

Alzheimer's Association Chapters

Alabama

Mid South Chapter, North Alabama Regional Office - 3222 S. Memorial Parkway, Century Office Center, Ste. 16. Bldg. 200, Huntsville, AL 35801 Huntsville URL: *http://www.jtsgraphics.com/alz/*

Arkansas

Central Arkansas Chapter - URL: *http://www.alzark.org/*

Oklahoma/Arkansas Chapter - 6465 South Yale, Suite 206, Tulsa, OK 74136 Phone: (918) 481-7741 URL: *http://www.alzokar.org/*

Western Arkansas Chapter - 320 North Greenwood Avenue, Fort Smith, AR 72901 URL: *http://www.alzokar.org/arkansas/*

Arizona

Desert Southwest Chapter - 1028 E. McDowell Road, Phoenix, AZ 85006 Phone: (602) 528-0545 or (800) 392-0022 URL: *http://www.alzaz.org/*

California

California Central Coast Chapter - 2024 De La Vina, Suite B, Santa Barbara, CA 93105 Phone: (805) 563-0020 or (800) 660-1993 URL: *http://www.centralcoastalz.org/*

Los Angeles, Riverside and San Bernardino Counties Chapter - 5900 Wilshire Blvd., Suite 1700, Los Angeles, CA 90036 Phone: (323) 938-3379 or (800) 660-1993 URL: *http://www.alzla.org/*

Northern California Chapter - 2065 West El Camino Real, Suite C, Mountain View, CA 94040 Phone: (650) 962-8111 or (800) 660-1993 URL: *http://www.alznorcal.org/*

Northern California Chapter, Greater Sacramento Area Chapter - URL: *http://www.sacalz.org/*

Orange County Chapter - 2540 N. Santiago Blvd., Orange, CA 92867 Phone: (714) 283-1111 or (800) 660-1993 URL: *http://www.alzoc.org/*

San Diego Chapter - 8514 Commerce Avenue, San Diego, CA 92121 Phone: (858) 537-5040 or (800) 660-1993 URL: *http://www.sanalz.org/index2.html*

Ventura County Chapter - URL: *http://www.alz.org/ventura/*

Colorado

Rocky Mountain Chapter - 789 Sherman Street, Suite 500, Denver, CO 80203 Phone: (303) 813-1669 or (800) 864-4404 URL: *http://www.alzrockymtn.org/*

Connecticut

Northern Connecticut Chapter - 96 Oak Street, Hartford, CT 06106 Phone: (860) 956-9560 or (800) 356-5502 URL: *http://www.alzct.org/*

Southern Connecticut Chapter - URL: *http://www.ctalz.org/*

Delaware

Delaware Valley Chapter - 100 N. 17th Street, 2nd Floor, Philadelphia, PA 19103 Phone: (215) 561-2919, (215) 561-4661 or (800) 272-3900 URL: *http://www.alz-delawarevalley.org/*

District of Columbia

National Capitol Chapter - URL: *http://www.alzheimersdc-md.org/*

Florida

Central and North Florida Chapter - 2010 Mizell Avenue, Winter Park, FL 32792 Phone: (407) 629-1997 URL: *http://www.alzorlando.org/*

Florida Gulf Coast/Tampa Bay Chapter - 9365 U.S. Hwy. 19 N., Suite B, Pinellas Park, FL 33782 Phone: (727) 578-2558 or (800) 772-8672 URL: *http://www.alz-tbc.org/*

Manatee/Sarasota Counties Chapter - URL: *http://www.alzswfl.org/*

South Florida Chapter - 1175 N.E. 125th. Street, Suite 600, Miami, FL 33161 Phone: (305) 891-6228

Southeast Florida Chapter - 8333 W. McNab Road, Suite 210, Fort Lauderdale, FL 33321 Phone: (954) 726-0002 or (800) 861-7826 URL: *http://www.alzsefc.org/*

Georgia

Georgia Chapter - 1925 Century Blvd, Suite 10, Atlanta, GA 30345 Phone: (404) 728-1181 or (888) 649-7800 URL: *http://www.alzga.org/*

Hawaii

Aloha Chapter - 1050 Ala Moana Blvd, Suite Bldg D, Honolulu, HI 96814 Phone: (808) 591-2771

Idaho

Oregon Greater Idaho Chapter - 1311 N.W. 21st Avenue, Portland, OR 97209 Phone: (503) 413-7115 or (800) 733-0402 URL: *http://www.alz.org/oregon/*

Illinois

Central Illinois Chapter - 606 W. Glen Avenue, Peoria, IL 61614 Phone: (309) 681-1100 or (800) 681-1181 URL: *http://www.alzillinois.org/*

Greater Illinois Chapter - 4709 Golf Road, Suite 1015, Skokie, IL 60076 Phone: (847) 933-2413 or (800) 272-3900 URL: *http://www.alzheimers-illinois.org/*

Indiana

Central Indiana Chapter - 9135 North Meridian Street, Suite B-4, Indianapolis, IN 46260 Phone: (800) 272-3900, (317) 575-9620 or (888) 575-9624 URL: *http://www.standbyyou.org/*

Greater Kentucky and Southern Indiana Chapter - 3703 Taylorsville Road, Suite 102, Louisville, KY 40220 Phone: (502) 451-4266 or (800) 221-1277 URL: *http://www.alzinky.org/*

Northern Indiana Chapter - 108 N Main Street, Suite 707, South Bend, IN 46601 Phone: (574) 232-4121 or (888) 303-0180 URL: *http://www.alz-nic.org/*

Iowa

Big Sioux Chapter - 522 4th Street, Lower Level, P. O. Box 3716 Sioux City, IA 51101 Phone: (712) 279-5802 or (800) 426-6512 URL: *http://www.alz-sioux.org/*

East Central Iowa Chapter - 1642 42nd Street N.E., Cedar Rapids, IA 52402 Phone: (319) 294-9699 or (888) 397-9635 URL: *http://www.alzeci.org/*

Greater Iowa Chapter - 700 E. University, Level B, Iowa Lutheran Hospital, Des Moines, IA - 50316 Phone: (515) 263-2464 or (800) 738-8071 URL: *http://www.alz.org/greateriowa/*

Kansas

Heart of America Chapter - 3846 West 75th Street, Prairie Village, KS 66208 Phone: (913) 831-3888 or (800) 733-1981 URL: *http://www.kcalz.org/*

Sunflower Chapter - 347 South Laura, Wichita, KS 67211 Phone: (316) 267-7333 or (877) 267-7333 URL: *http://www.alzheimerskansas.org/*

Kentucky

Greater Kentucky and Southern Indiana Chapter - 3703 Taylorsville Road, Suite 102, Louisville, KY 40220 Phone: (502) 451-4266 or (800) 221-1277 URL: *http://www.alzinky.org/*

Louisiana

Greater New Orleans Chapter - 1040 Calhoun Street, New Orleans, LA 70118 Phone: (504) 895-6223 or (800) 459-3528

North East Louisiana Chapter - P. O. Box 2471, Monroe, LA 71207 Phone: (318) 322-2828 or (888) 202-2828 URL: *http://www.bayou.com/alzheimers/*

Maine

Maine Chapter - 163 Lancaster St., Suite 160B, Portland, ME 04101 Phone: (207) 772-0115 or (800) 660-2871 URL: *http://www.mainealz.org/*

Maryland

Greater Maryland Chapter - 1850 York Road, Suite D, Lutherville Timonium, MD - 21093 Phone: (410) 561-9099 or (800) 443-2273 URL: *http://www.alzcmd.org/*

National Capitol Area Chapter - 11240 Waples Mill Road, Suite 402, Fairfax, VA Phone: (866) 259-0042 or (866) 259-0042 URL: *http://www.alz-nca.org/*

Western Maryland Chapter - URL: *http://www.alzwmd.org/*

Massachusetts

Massachusetts Chapter - 36 Cameron Avenue, Cambridge, MA 02140 Phone: (617) 868-6718 or (800) 548-2111 URL: *http://www.alzmass.org/*

Michigan

Greater Michigan Chapter - 17220 West 12 Mile Road, Suite 100, Southfield, MI 48076 Phone: (248) 557-8277 or (800) 337-3827 URL: *http://www.alzgmc.org/*

Michigan Great Lakes Chapter - 107 Aprill Dr. Suite 1, Ann Arbor, MI 48103 Phone: (734) 677-3081 or (800) 337-3827 URL: *http://www.alzmigreatlakes.org/*

North/West Michigan Chapter - 225 W. 30th Street, Holland, MI 49423 Phone: (616) 392-8365 or (800) 893-8365 URL: *http://www.nwmialz.org/*

West Michigan Chapter - URL: *http://www.alzheimers-westmi.org/*

Minnesota

Minnesota-Dakotas Chapter - 4550 W. 77th Street, Suite 200, Minneapolis, MN 55435 Phone: (952) 830-0512 or (800) 232-0851 URL: *http://www.alzmn.org/*

Mississippi

Mississippi Chapter - 1900 Dunbarton Drive, Suite Interstate, Jackson, MS 39216 Phone: (601) 987-0020 or (877) 525-HELP

Missouri

Mid-Missouri Chapter - 1121 Business Loop 70 East, Suite 2B, Columbia, MO 65201 Phone: (573) 443-8665 or (800) 693-8665

Southwest Missouri Chapter - 1500 S. Glenstone, Glen Isle Center, Springfield, MO 65804 Phone: (417) 886-2199 or (800) 487-0747

St. Louis Chapter - 9374 Olive Boulevard, Saint Louis, MO 63132 Phone: (314) 432-3422 or (800) 980-9080 URL: *http://www.alzstl.org/*

Montana

Montana Chapter - 2900 12th Avenue, Suite 4E, Billings, MT 59101 Phone: (406) 252-3053 URL: *http://www.alz-mt.org/*

Nebraska

Great Plains Chapter - 5601 S. 27th Street, Suite 201, Lincoln, NE 68512 Phone: (402) 420-2540 or (800) 487-2585 URL: *http://www.alznebraska.org/*

Midlands/Omaha and Eastern Nebraska Chapter - 7101 Newport Avenue, Suite 305, Omaha, NE 68152 Phone: (402) 572-3059 or (800) 309-2112 URL: *http://www.omaha-cb-alz.org/*

Nevada

Desert Southwest Chapter - 1028 E. McDowell Road, Phoenix, AZ 85006 Phone: (602) 528-0545 or (800) 392-0022 URL: *http://www.alzaz.org/*

Northern California and Northern Nevada Chapter - 2065 West El Camino Real, Suite C, Mountain View, CA 94040 Phone: (650) 962-8111 or (800) 660-1993 URL: *http://www.alznorcal.org/*

New Hampshire

Vermont and New Hampshire Chapter - 338 River Street, Montpelier, VT 05601 Phone: (603) 226-5868 or (800) 536-8864 URL: *http://www.alz.org/vtnh/*

New Jersey

Greater New Jersey Chapter - 400 Morris Avenue, Suite 251, Denville, NJ 07834 Phone: (973) 586-4300 or (800) 883-1180 URL: *http://www. alz.org/chapters/template/njersey/*

New Mexico

New Mexico Chapter - 8100 Mountain Road NE, Suite 201, Albuquerque, NM 87110 Phone: (505) 266-4473 or (800) 777-8155 URL: *http://www. nm-alzheimers.org/*

New York

Central New York Chapter - 441 West Kirkpatrick Street, Syracuse, NY 13204 Phone: (315) 472-4201 or (800) 339-4177 URL: *http://www.alzcny.org/*

Hudson Valley/Rockland/Westchester Chapter - 2 Jefferson Plaza, Suite 203, Poughkeepsie, NY 12601 Phone: (845) 471-2655 or (800) 872-0994 URL: *http://www.alzhudsonvalley.org/*

Long Island Chapter - 3281 Veteran's Memorial Highway, Suite E-13, Ronkonkoma, NY 11779 Phone: (631) 580-5100 URL: *http://www. alzheimersli.org/*

New York City Chapter - 360 Lexington Avenue, 5th Floor, New York, NY 10017 Phone: (212) 983-0700 URL: *http://www.alzheimernyc.org/*

Northeastern New York Chapter - 85 Watervliet Avenue, Albany, NY 12206 Phone: (518) 438-2217 or (800) 303-2218 URL: *http://www.alzneny.org/site/home.asp*

Rochester Chapter - 435 East Henrietta Road, Rochester, NY 14620 Phone: (585) 760-5400 or (800) 724-0587 URL: *http://www.alz-rochesterny.org/*

Southern Tier Chapter URL: *http://www.alz.org/chapters/template/sothtier/Welcome.html*

Western New York Chapter - 1284 French Road, Depew, NY 14043 Phone: (716) 656-8448 or (800) 273-6737 URL: *http://www.alzwny.org/working/home/home.htm*

North Carolina

Eastern North Carolina Chapter - 400 Oberlin Road, Suite 208, Raleigh, NC 27605 Phone: (919) 832-3732 or (800) 228-8738 URL: *http://www.alznc.org/*

Western Carolina Chapter - 3800 Shamrock Drive, Charlotte, NC 28215 Phone: (704) 532-7390, (704) 532-7392 or (800) 888-6671 URL: *http://www.perigee.net/~alz/*

North Dakota

Minnesota-Dakotas Chapter - 4550 W. 77th Street, Suite 200, Minneapolis, MN 55435 Phone: (952) 830-0512 or (800) 232-0851 URL: *http://www.alzmn.org/*

Ohio

Central Ohio Chapter - 3380 Tremont Road, Columbus, OH 43221 Phone: (614) 457-6003 or (800) 735-6751

Cleveland Area Chapter - 12200 Fairhill Road, Cleveland, OH 44120 Phone: (216) 721-8457 or (800) 441-3322

East Central Ohio Chapter - 126 W. Church Street, Newark, OH 43055 Phone: (740) 345-5102 or (800) 441-3322

Greater Cincinnati Chapter - 644 Linn Street, Suite 1026, Cincinnati, OH 45203 Phone: (513) 721-4284 or (800) 441-3322 URL: *http://www.alz.org/grtrcinc/*

Greater East Ohio Chapter - 1815 West Market Street, Suite 301, Akron, OH 44313 Phone: (330) 864-5646 or (800) 441-3322 URL: *http://www. tricountyalz.org/*

Miami Valley Chapter - 3797 Summit Glen Drive, Suite G100, The Laurelwood, Dayton, OH 45449 Phone: (937) 291-3332 or (800) 441-3322

Northwest Ohio Chapter - 2500 N. Reynolds Road, Toledo, OH 43615 Phone: (419) 537-1999 (800) 441-3322 URL: *http://www.nwoalz.org/*

Oklahoma

Oklahoma Chapter - 6465 South Yale, Suite 206, Tulsa, OK 74136 Phone: (918) 481-7741 or (800) 493-1411 URL: *http://www.alzokar.org/oklahoma/*

Oregon

Oregon Greater Idaho Chapter - 1311 N.W. 21st Avenue, Portland, OR 97209 Phone: (503) 413-7115 or (800) 733-0402 URL: *http://www.alz.org/oregon/*

Southern Oregon Chapter - URL: *http://id.mind.net/community/alzheimers/alzstart.htm*

Pennsylvania

Delaware Valley Chapter - 100 N. 17th Street, 2nd Floor, Philadelphia, PA 19103 Phone: (215) 561-2919, (215) 561-4661 or (800) 272-3900 URL: *http://www. alz-delawarevalley.org/*

Greater Pennsylvania Chapter - 2001 North Front Street, Suite 321, Building 2, Harrisburg, PA 17102 Phone: (717) 232-3580 or (800) 975-8848

Rhode Island

Rhode Island Chapter - 245 Waterman Street, Suite 306, Providence, RI 02906 Phone: (401) 421-0008 or (800) 244-1428 URL: *http://www.alz-ri.org/*

South Carolina

Palmetto Chapter - P. O. Box 7044, Columbia, SC 29202 Phone: (803) 772-3346 or (800) 636-3346 URL: *http://www.midnet.sc.edu/alz/alz.htm*

South Dakota

Minnesota/Dakotas Chapter - 4550 W. 77th Street, Suite 200, Minneapolis, MN 55435 Phone: (952) 830-0512 or (800) 232-0851 URL: *http://www. alzmndak.org/*

Tennessee

Eastern Tennessee Chapter - 2200 Sutherland Avenue, Portland Building, Suite H 102, Knoxville, TN 37919 Phone: (865) 544-6288 URL: *http://www. tnalz.org/*

Mid-South Chapter - 4004 Hillsboro Pike, Suite 219B, Nashville, TN 37215 Phone: (615) 292-4938 URL: *http://www.alztn.org/*

Northeast Tennessee Chapter - 207 N. Boone Street, Suite 1500, Johnson City, TN 37604 Phone: (423) 928-4080

Southeast Tennessee Chapter - 735 Broad Street, Suite 300, Chattanooga, TN 37402 Phone: (423) 265-3600 Phone: (800) 616-1922

Texas

Greater Austin Chapter - 3420 Executive Center Drive, Suite 301, Austin, TX 78731 Phone: (512) 241-0420 or (800) 367-2132 URL: *http://www. alz-austin.org/*

Greater Dallas Chapter - 7610 Stemmons, Suite 600, Dallas, TX 75247 Phone: (214) 827-0062, (214) 540-2400 or (800) 515-8201 URL: *http://www.alzdallas.org/*

Houston and Southeast Texas Chapter - 11251 Northwest Freeway, Suite 300, Houston, TX 77092 Phone: (713) 266-6400 or (800) 266-8744 URL: *http://www.alztex.org/*

North Central Texas Chapter - P. O. Box 9709, Fort Worth, TX 76147 Phone: (817) 336-4949 or (800) 471-4422 URL: *http://www.alz.org/northcentraltexas/*

Star Chapter - 4400 N. Mesa, Suite 9, El Paso, TX 79902 Phone: (915) 544-1799 or (877) 544-1799

Utah

Utah Chapter - 1414 E. 4500 South, Suite 2, Salt Lake City, UT 84117 Phone: (801) 274-1944 or (800) 371-6694 URL: *http://www.alzutah.org/*

Vermont

Vermont and New Hampshire Chapter - 338 River Street, Montpelier, VT 05601 Phone: (603) 226-5868 or (800) 536-8864 URL: *http://www.alz.org/vtnh/*

Virginia

Blue Ridge of Virginia Chapter - URL: *http://www.alzblueridge.org/*

Central and Western Virginia Chapter - P. O. Box 4634, Charlottesville, VA 22905 Phone: (434) 973-6122 or (888) 809-7383

Greater Richmond Chapter - 4600 Cox Road, Suite 130, Glen Allen, VA 23060 Phone: (804) 967-2580 or (800) 598-4673 URL: *http://www.richmondalzheimers.org/*

National Capitol Area Chapter - 11240 Waples Mill Road, Suite 402, Fairfax, VA 22030 Phone: (866) 259-0042 URL: *http://www.alz-nca.org/*

Southeastern Virginia Chapter - #20 Interstate Corporate Center, Suite 233, Norfolk, VA 23502 Phone: (757) 459-2405 or (800) 755-1129

Washington

Inland Northwest Chapter - 601 W. Maxwell #4, Spokane, WA 99201 Phone: (509) 483-8456 or (800) 256-6659 URL: *http://www.inwalz.org/*

Western and Central Washington State Chapter - 12721 30th Avenue N.E., Suite 101, Seattle, WA 98125 Phone: (206) 363-5500 or (800) 848-7097 URL: *http://www.alzwa.org/*

West Virginia

West Virginia Chapter - 1111 Lee Street East, Charleston, WV 25301 Phone: (304) 343-2717 or (800) 491-2717 URL: *http://wvalzheimers.homestead.com/wvalzheimersmain.html*

Wisconsin

Greater Wisconsin Chapter - 2900 Curry Lane, Suite A, Green Bay, WI 54311 Phone: (920) 469-2110 or (800) 360-2110

South Central Wisconsin Chapter - 517 N. Segoe, Suite 301, Madison, WI 53705 Phone: (608) 232-3400 or (800) 428-9280 URL: *http://www.alzwisc.org/*

Southeastern Wisconsin Chapter - 6130 W. National Avenue, Suite 200, Milwaukee, WI 53214 Phone: (414) 479-8800 or (800) 922-2413 URL: *http://www.alzheimers-sewi.org/*

Wyoming

Great Plains Chapter - 5601 S. 27th Street, Suite 201, Lincoln, NE 68512 Phone: (402) 420-2540 or (800) 487-2585 URL: *http://www.alzgreatplains.org/*

APPENDIX C

Alzheimer's Organizations Worldwide

Alzheimer's Disease International - Alzheimer's Disease International, 45-46 Lower Marsh, London SE1 7RG UK Phone: +44 20 7620 3011 URL: *http://www.alz.co.uk/*

Argentina

Asociación de Lucha contra el Mal de Alzheimer - Lacarra No 78 1407 Capital Federal, Buenos Aires, Argentina Phone: +54 11 4671 1187 URL: *http://www.alma-alzheimer.org.ar/*

Australia

Alzheimer's Association of Tasmania - 169 Campbell Street, Hobart 7000, Tasmania Australia Phone: 002 348444 or 1800 639 331 URL: *http://www.tased.edu.au/tasonline/tasalz/tasalz.htm*

Alzheimer's Association of Western Australia - P. O. Box 1509, Subiaco, WA 6904 Phone: 08 9388 2800 or 1800-639-331 URL: *http://www.alzheimers.asn.au/*

Alzheimer's Association Victoria - 98-104 Riversdale Road, Locked Bag 3001, Hawthorn, Victoria 3122, Australia 03 9815 7800 or 1800 639 331 URL: *http://www.alzvic.asn.au/index.htm*

Alzheimer's Australia New South Wales - P. O. Box 6042, North Ryde, NSW 1670, Australia Phone: 02 9805 0100 or 1800 639 331 URL:*http://www. alznsw.asn.au/*

Austria

Alzheimer Angehorige Austria - Obere Augartenstrasse 26-28 1020 Vienna, Austria Phone: +43 1 332 5166 URL: *http://www.alzheimer-selbsthilfe.at/*

Belgium

Ligue Alzheimer - Clinique Le Perî, 4B Rue Montagne Sainte Walburge B-4000 Liège Phone: +32 4 225 8793 URL: *http://www.alzheimer.be/*

Brazil

Associaco Brasilier de Alzheimer - Caixa Postal 3913, São Paulo, SP Cep 01060-970 Phone: 0800 55 1906 URL: *http://www.abraz.com.br/*

Canada

Alzheimer's Society of Canada - 20 Eglinton Ave. W., Ste. 1200, Toronto, ON M4R 1K8 Phone: (416)488-8772 or (800) 616-8816 URL: *http://www. alzheimer.ca/*

Alzheimer's Society Toronto - Alzheimer Society of Toronto 2323 Yonge Street, Suite 500, Toronto, ON M4P 2C9 Phone: (416) 322-6560 URL: *http://www.asmt.org/*

China

Chinese Association of Alzheimer's Disease and Related Disorders - Department of Neurology, Beijing Hospital, Ministry of Health #1 Da Hua Road, Dong Dan Beijing 100730, China Phone: +8610 6521 2012 Email: *xuxh@public.bta.net.cn*

Chile

Corporación Chilena de la Enfermedad, de Alzheimer y Afecciones Similares - Desiderio Lemus 0143 Recoleta Santiago, Chile Phone: +56 2 236 0846 Email: *alzchile@mi.terra.cl*

Columbia

Asociacion Colombiana de Alzheimer y Desordenes Relacionados - Calle 69 A No. 10-16 Santafe deBogota D.C. Colombia Phone: +57 1 348 1997 Email: *alzheimercolombia@hotmail.com*

Costa Rica

Alzheimer's Association of Costa Rica - Apartado 4755 San José 1000 Costa Rica Phone: +506 290 28 44 Email: *ximajica@sol.racsa.co.cr*

Cuba

Cuban Section of Alzheimer's Disease and Related Disorders - Calle 146 No 2504 e/ 25 y 31 Cubanacan Playa Ciudad de la Habana Cuba Phone: +537 220974 Fax: +537 336857 Email: *inmo@teleda.get.tur.cu*

Cyprus

Pancyprian Association of Alzheimer's Disease - 31A Stadiou 6020 Larnaca Cyprus Phone: +357 4 627 104 Fax: +357 4 627 106 Email: *alzhcyprus@yahoo.com*

Czech Republic

Ceska Alzheimerovska Spolecnost Centre of Gerontology - Simunkova 1600 18200 Praha 8 Czech Republic Phone: +420 2 88 36 76 Email: *Petr.Veleta@gerontocentrum.cz*

Denmark

Alzheimerforeningen - Sankt Lukas Vej 6,1 DK-2900, Hellerup Denmark Phone: +45-39-40 04 88 URL: *http://www.alzheimer.dk/*

Europe

Alzheimer Europe - URL: *http://www.alzheimer-europe.org/*

Finland

Alzheimer-keskusliitto ry - Luotsikatu 4 E, 00160 Helsinki, Finland Phone: +358-9-622 62 00 URL: *http://www.alzheimer.fi/*

France

Association France Alzheimer - 23 rue Gabriel Beaumarié 45240 LA FERTÉ ST AUBIN (Loiret) Phone: 02 38 64 88 22 URL: *http://www.francealzheimer.com/*

Germany

Deutsche Alzheimer Gesellschaft e.V. - Friedrichstr. 236, D-10969 Berlin, Germany Phone: +49-30-31 50 57 33 URL: *http://www.deutsche-alzheimer.de/*

Ireland

Western Alzheimer Foundation - Mount Street, Claremorris, Co Mayo, Ireland Phone: +353 94 62480 URL: *http://www.connect.ie/users/waf/*

Italy

Alzheimer Italia - Via T.Marino, 7 - 20121 Milano Phone: 02-809767 r.a. URL: *http://www.geocities.com/HotSprings/1420/*

Mexico

Asociación Alzheimer de Monterrey - URL: *http://www.geocities.com/HotSprings/Spa/7712/entrada.html*

Netherlands

Alzheimer Nederland - URL: *http://www.alzheimer-ned.nl/*

Pakistan

Alzheimer's Pakistan -146/1 Shadman Jail Road, Lahore 54000, Pakistan Phone: +92 42 759 6589 URL: *http://www.alz.org.pk/*

Philippines

ADAP - St Luke's Medical Center, Medical Arts Bldg, Rm. 410, E Rodriguez Sr Avenue, Quezon City, Philippines Phone: 632 723 1039 URL: *http://www.alzphilippines.com/*

Poland

Polish Alzheimer's Association - ul.Hoza, 54/1 00-682 Warszawa, Poland, Phone: + 48 22 622 11 22 URL: *http://www.alzheimer.pl/intro.html*

Puerto Rica

Asociación de Alzheimer de P.R. - Apartado 362026, San Juan, Puerto Rico 00936-2026 Phone: +1 787 727 4151 URL: *http://www.alzheimerpr.org/*

Romania

Romanian Alzheimer Society - Bd.Mihail Kogalniceanu 95A, Sc. A. Et.1, Ap. 8, Sector 5, Bucharest, Romania 70603 Phone: +40 1 686 3470 URL: *http://www.alzheimer-europe.org/Romania/*

Scotland

Alzheimer Scotland, Action on Dementia - 22 Drumsheugh Gardens, Edinburgh, EH3 7RN, Scotland Phone: +44 131 243 1453 URL: *http://www.alzscot.org/*

Singapore

Alzheimer's Disease Association - Blk 157, Toa Payoh, Lorong 1, #01- 1195, Singapore 310157 Phone: +65 353 8734 URL: *http://www.alzheimers.org.sg/*

Spain

Confederación Española de Familiares de Enfermos de Alzheimer - Avda Pio XII, 37, Entreplanta, Oficina 5, 31008 Pamplona, Spain Phone: +34 948 177 907 URL: *http://www.ceafa.org/*

Sweden

Alzheimerföreningen i Sverige - Sunnanväg 14 S, 222 26 Lund, Sweden Phone: +46 46 14 73 18 URL: *http://www.alzheimerforeningen.nu/*

Switzerland

Association Alzheimer Suisse - 8 Rue des Pêcheurs, CH-1400 Yverdon-les-Bains, Switzerland Phone: +41 24 426 2000 URL: *http://www.alz.ch/*

Thailand

Alzheimer's and Related Disorders Association of Thailand - 114 Pinakorn 4, Boramratchachunee Road, Talingchan, Bangkok 10170, Thailand Phone: +66 2 880 8542/7539 URL: *http://www.geocities.com/alzheimerasso/*

Turkey

Turkish Alzheimer Society - Alzheimer Vakfi, Lamartin Cad. Celik Palak, Apt. No: 44/11 Taksim, Istanbul, Turkey Phone: +90 212 2563370 URL: *http://www.medyatext.com/alzheimer/*

United Kingdom

Alzheimer's Society - Gordon House,10 Greencoat Place, London SW1P 1PH United Kingdom URL: *http://www.alzheimers.org.uk/*

Venezeula

Fundación Alzheimer de Venezuela - Av. El Limón, Qta. Mi Muñe, El Cafetal, Caracas Phone: +58 212 4146129 URL: *http://www.mujereslegendarias.org.ve/alzheimer.htm*

Appendix D

Book Sources

Topic-Specific Bookstores

AD/Caregiving Bookstore - URL:
http://www.vstore.com/cgi-bin/pagegen/vstorereading/adcaregiving/

Ageless Design Alzheimer's Store - URL:
http://www.thealzheimersstore.com/

AlzBrain.org Alzheimer's Videos - URL:
http://www.alzbrain.org/resource/videos.html

Alzheimer's Disease Bookstore - URL:
http://www.wellnessbooks.com/alzheimers/

Elder Books - URL: *http://www.elderbooks.com/*

ElderCare Bookstore - URL:
http://www.ec-online.net/Connections/bookstore.htm

HeartSong Books - URL: *http://heartsongbooks.com/carebook.html*

A Place for the Humanities Alzheimer's Bookstore - URL: *http://www.geocities.com/SoHo/Coffeehouse/3321/adbookstore.html*

Suite101 Alzheimer's Disease Topic Library - URL:
http://www.suite101.com/books.cfm/15157

Top Alzheimer's Caregiving Sites Book Shop - URL:
http://communities.iuniverse.com/bin/bookshop.asp?circleid=6622

Major Bookstores

Amazon - URL:
http://www.amazon.com/exec/obidos/tg/browse/-/760792/002-3821440-6562461

Barnes & Noble - URL:
http://search.barnesandnoble.com/booksearch/results.asp?WRD=alzheimer

Books-a-Million - URL:
http://www.booksamillion.com/ncom/books?id=2322284767902

Out-of-Print Dealers

Alibris - URL: *http://www.alibris.com/*

Powell's - URL: *http://www.powells.com/*

Price Comparison Tools

Add-All - URL: *http://www.addall.com/*

AllBookstores.com - URL: *http://www.allbookstores.com/*

BookBrain.uk - URL: *http://www.bookbrain.co.uk/*

BookHQ - URL: *http://www.bookhq.com/*

BookPrices.com - URL: *http://www.bookprices.com/*

Bublos - URL: *http://www.bublos.com/*

EveryBookstore.com - URL: *http://ebs.allbookstores.com/*

ISBN.nu - URL: *http://isbn.nu/*

MySimon - URL:
http://www.mysimon.com/category/index.jhtml?c=bookisbn&v=1

Libraries

Alzheimer's Association's Benjamin B. Green-Field Library - URL:
http://www.alz.org/ResourceCenter/Programs/LibraryServices.htm

Alzheimer's Society of Canada's Library - URL:
http://www.alzheimer.ca/english/resources/library-intro.htm

Gateway to Library Catalogs at the Library of Congress - URL:
http://lcweb.loc.gov/z3950/gateway.html#lc

Library of Congress Online Catalog - URL: *http://catalog.loc.gov/*

LibWeb: Library Servers via the WWW - URL:
http://sunsite.berkeley.edu/Libweb/

0-595-25356-3